☐ Read 4,6,7

# Yoga and Ayurveda

*An Evolutionary Approach*

PAUL DUGLISS, M.D.

No part of this book is intended to substitute for medical advice, diagnosis, or treatment. Every individual is unique, and no book can possibly address each person's special situation. Do not make changes in your medications or lifestyle without consulting your health care provider. The information contained in this book is intended to stimulate discussion with your health care providers and not to replace their advice.

ISBN 978-0-9721233-2-7

*For all seekers...*

# Acknowledgements

I do not claim to be the originator of these ideas. The great seers and the great saints of modern time such as Maharishi Mahesh Yogi, Maharishi Sadashiva Isham, Elizabeth Haich, Charlie Lutes and many others are all owed the honor of restoring this timeless knowledge. My role is to be the conveyer of this knowledge and to serve as a conduit for the revolutionizing of our ideas about health and healing. I owe a great debt to all my students for inspiring this book, and to the love and support of family and friends who have made my work in this world possible.

10

# CONTENTS

# Yoga and Ayurveda

*Chapter 1*

PURPOSE

# Purpose

No greater confusion exists than the relationship between Yoga and Ayurveda. Lost in the millennia, the essence of this knowledge is now in a state of revival. The fragmentation in the collective consciousness that has so divided the world into factions and religions and political parties is clearly represented in the common view of the relationship of Yoga and Ayurveda. The time has come for the fragmented approach to life to fall by the wayside and make room for the integrated wholeness that is the essence of life itself. The understanding of this ancient wisdom has been so lost that Yoga and Ayurveda are viewed as separate disciplines, each with its own tradition and philosophy. Nothing could be further from the truth.

The illusion of separateness is fostered by a lack of understanding of the nature of consciousness and the universe. The fundamental truths that the ancients elucidated can only be understood by comprehending the level of the enlightened. It is the sad history of the world that the enlightened have spoken from their level and the unenlightened have heard from theirs. Thus, knowledge gets distorted and misinterpreted and turned from a practical overview into either an intellectual exercise or into a set of rules that are adhered to with fundamentalist fervor.

Fortunately for us, this is a time when the knowledge of life and reality is being transformed from all sides — from physics and science, to religion, to everyday language. As more and more people get a "feel" for the vastness and orderliness of spiritual reality and let go of the illusion that we are just isolated little egos within bags of skin, the level of the enlightened becomes easier to grasp. New concepts of consciousness and connectedness are easily assimilated. New ways of thinking about "coincidence" and possibility are emerging in all areas of society. This new way of thinking allows the mechanics of consciousness to be more readily accepted. With these concepts within reach of the unenlightened, the expressions and descriptions emanating from the enlightened become comprehensible.

In order to understand the relationship between Yoga and Ayurveda, we must understand the nature of consciousness — what it is, how it works, how it relates to healing and to the practices of Yoga. To even understand the purpose of Ayurveda or the purpose of Yoga we must understand consciousness. The ancients, Charaka and Patanjali, have given clear descriptions of the purpose of each. Charaka was the first to "canonize" Ayurveda. He was the ancient internist extraordinaire, as opposed to Sushruta, the famous surgeon who performed more than 60 types of operations on the eye alone, was able to reattach severed limbs, and whose surgical instruments became the design for many modern surgical tools.

Charaka was the first to outline a set of aphorisms — a set of verses initially passed down as an oral tradition, and only written down years later. What is important to understand is that Charaka clearly states that the knowledge he presents is not his own. His first aphorisms describe the knowledge as being cognized by ancient seers in meditation. As part of the first book of aphorisms, Charaka explicitly lays out the purpose of Ayurveda. This is presented below from two different translations. And, thus, the trouble begins:

> Mind, soul, and body, this trinity, called person, resteth on union like three sticks (standing with one another's support). Upon that (trinity) everything rests. That is also called *purusha* or being. It is also animate. That is regarded as the subject matter of this Science; and it is also for the sake of that, that this Science is promulgated.
>
> — *Charaka Samhita*
> *Kaviratna Translation*

3

> Mind, soul, and body — these three are like a tripod; the world is sustained by their combination; they constitute the substratum for everything. This (combination of the above three) is *Purusha*; this is sentient and this is the subject matter of this *Veda* (Ayurveda); it is for this that this *Veda* (Ayurveda) is brought to light.
>
> — *Charaka Samhita*
> *Sharma/Dash Translation*

Look at the first two sentences of the first translation. Note that the words in parentheses are added by the translator as a way of clarifying the translation. What is clearly being explained is that mind, soul and body rest on something that "everything" rests on. What is it that everything rests on? It is "being" or what is called *purusha* in Vedic terminology. So when Charaka says, "Upon that everything rests" what he is referring to as "that" is "being" or *purusha* and not, as the translator suggests in parentheses, on "trinity." Obviously, the "trinity" is what makes up a living person and there would be no need for Charaka to describe it as animate or sentient, if he were referring to "trinity." He's not. He is referring to that upon which the trinity rests. That underlying field of being out of which all creation arises is "animate." And *"that"* is the subject matter of Ayurveda.

So what is it that underlies mind, soul and body? What is it that underlies all of creation? What is this being or *purusha*? If that is the subject of the next four volumes of sayings of Charaka, we need to have a clear understanding. And note how far the second translation strays. Without a concept of an underlying field of being, the translator describes *purusha* as the combination of mind, soul and body, which even Yoga teachers in the West would recognize as a misuse of the term *purusha*. "Being" is not composed of mind, soul and body — it *underlies* them.

4

In this manner, without a proper insight into the intention of the seers, without an understanding of how the universe works, it is easy to misconstrue the purpose of Ayurveda and get lost in thinking it is about the unity of mind, soul and body.

In order to understand Ayurveda and Yoga, we must understand what consciousness is, what being is and how all of creation arises out of one underlying field of energy and intelligence. If there is anything that the quantum physicists are trying to tell us about reality, it is this:

*There is an underlying field of vast energy and organizing power that underlies all material creation.*

That being reality, all our energy and liveliness arises out of that field as well. All of "us" comes from "that." And all of Ayurveda is about "that." In other words, if we can understand how mind, soul and body arise out of this underlying field and are support by it, then we can understand how to influence, change and transform our existence — we can understand how to create health and how to heal.

If all that we are arises out of one underlying field of energy and intelligence, then our sense of ourselves and being separate from others and separate from almighty Nature is an illusion and a hoax. Then, indeed, this "being" becomes a subject worthy of study. To understand what Charaka was saying we must have a better feel for this "being" or for what we will call consciousness. This consciousness model, by its very nature, challenges our illusions of ourselves.

## The Consciousness Model

What follows is a model for the reality. In that model, the body is more than a physical system. It is also an energetic system. Even beyond energies, there is a field out of which energy arises. That is what modern physicists are telling us. Given this, the body is not just energy. We are more complex than that, more intelligent, more organized. This model provides a way to set common illusions aside and understand reality and how we heal — the reality that Charaka and Patanjali both understood.

### We are Nonmaterial Beings

This model is one that makes use of some scientific facts to point to the big picture. In the grand scheme of any given life, the body is really a fleeting event. If you have the assumption that you *are* your body, that your cells have somehow gotten together and created a mind and a soul, then you have to know you were not here a year ago. Consider these facts:

- 98% of the molecules that make up the body are replaced in one year's time. The lining of the stomach replaces itself in five days.
- Liver cells are constantly being destroyed and replaced. Cut off a lobe of the liver, and it can replace itself in two months.
- Even the most solid part of us, our skeletal system, gets replaced continuously. Bone is constantly being reabsorbed and rebuilt. Osteoporosis is then the end result when there is an imbalance within this regeneration process.

Given these facts, the person you saw in the mirror this morning was not there a year ago. The body has been almost entirely replaced. Even brain cells, once thought not to regenerate, are constantly replacing their internal structure, if not creating new dendrites and losing old ones. The body is impermanent, yet we still persist. The only logical conclusion is that we are not just our physical bodies.

Another way to reach this understanding is to look at human memory. The human brain contains within it approximately 100 billion neurons. Yet despite this enormously vast number, we know these cells are highly organized in terms of their function. The cells at the back of the brain, for instance, relate to visual functions and to the processes responsible for sight, while large areas of the brain relate to movement and balance. However, even if the entire brain were utilized just for memory, it would still not be sufficient to store all the data that an average human can maintain and access.

Even the most sophisticated compression schemes to store data (such as is used to store movies on DVDs) are unable to compact information small enough for us to "fit" all that we know and can remember into the human brain. So where is it stored?

The only logical conclusion is that it is not stored in the brain. But if not in the brain, then where? Consider the possibility that the information does not reside in the brain but in a field of energy and intelligence that the brain can access.

**The Underlying Field**

The ever-changing nature of the body, and the concept of the brain as being insufficient to contain all our memories, gives rise to a fundamental shift in our thinking about who we are. The brain is not a complex computer that stores and creates thoughts. Logically, this is not possible. Instead, the brain functions to amplify signals from an underlying field. The brain is like an amplifier in your radio. You select a certain station to tune into — for instance, a certain thought — and this is amplified or brought to awareness. Because we know the brain can perceive a single photon or a single quantum of green light, we know the brain can operate on the quantum mechanical level. The nervous system is able to amplify things from a quantum level and create out of them an impression or thought.

This means that that which makes us uniquely human has nothing to do with the material world. The human being is essentially *not* a physical being. Everyone knows that a corpse, while still possessing all the parts of a living body, is not the same as a live human being. Even if we cause the dead body's lungs to move and stimulate its heart to beat with drugs, it is different from a living being who is on a respirator. So how do we objectively know the difference?

One of the criteria that helps doctors determine if someone on a respirator is dead is the electrical activity of the brain. A fundamental difference in brainwave activity exists in a living human being, which points out the fact we are essentially energetic beings who utilize energy and information contained in an underlying field. This is a profoundly different view from the modern medical one that focuses on the physical and chemical structure of the body. This model of the human being goes far beyond simple physical events in attempting to explain wholeness, health and healing.

If we are all just energy in the same field, how come we have the sense of being isolated and separate from other people? The field that underlies all energy and all life is the field of consciousness. And consciousness is a field that is alive. It must be. If everything arises from it, then life arises from it as well. Think of it like an ocean. The underlying field of energy and intelligence that forms and organizes creation has much diversity among its waves on the surface of the water.

If one "wave" is only aware of itself to the depth of 2 feet, then it feels separate. It does not perceive the connection between one wave and another. Suppose an individual wave named Fred is somehow able to become aware of the underlying pool of water that makes up the ocean and starts to sense some of the smaller flows and vibrations that are affecting the next crest over. Suddenly, Fred is able to get some impressions of what his fellow wave is experiencing.

Fred has become a "psychic" wave. All psychic and intuitive phenomena arise because consciousness is not limited to the edge of the physical body. Consciousness is a field that underlies all of creation.

In this manner, we are individual beings, nonmaterial and independent, yet connected, as we are all part of the same pool, the same ocean. What is the water? The water is consciousness. Our consciousness is that which is connected to a sea of consciousness and that sea contains tremendous energy, information and intelligence.

The model of the human being described in Ayurvedic medicine *is* a model of consciousness. At the base of the sea of consciousness, there are no waves, just stillness. On the surface, waves and vibrations form. Like any vibration, these are composed of different frequencies.

What do these different frequencies represent? Human physiology is essentially designed for the transformation of these various frequencies to create our thoughts, feelings and the energy that informs our physical being, as well as our awareness of them. Consciousness is like a white light, and the human being is like a prism. We transform energy and create various colors through various energy centers in the body.

Perhaps a more accurate analogy is electricity as it comes from the source, the power plant. At 100,000 volts, the electricity from its source would fry any electrical device in your home. As the electrical energy travels from the power station to your home and ultimately to an outlet to power your kitchen blender, the energy is down-regulated at various substations as it makes this journey. So the voltage, which began at 100,000 volts from the power plant, becomes just 120 volts by the time it reaches your home.

Like the power plant, consciousness at its source has tremendous power. Unlike electricity, though, it contains the intelligence for the many forms it inhabits. The various aspects of human existence such as the spirit, mind, emotions or the body, are the expressions of the various frequencies of consciousness. Just like a prism and the frequencies of light that form different colors, our entire existence is organized around transforming energy and consciousness into the human experience: "Mind, soul, and body resteth on that."

**Three Basic Principles**

Three important principles are to be derived from the consciousness model:

- Whenever the flow of consciousness and its intelligence and energy are blocked, the potential for disorganization and disease is created.

- Health is re-created when contact is made with the source of consciousness. This reconnection re-establishes wholeness in the individual.

- Consciousness is a creative force. Just as a garden grows when we nourish and maintain it, our consciousness enlivens as we apply awareness to specific areas of it.

Health is maintained and nurtured by the frictionless flow of energy and intelligence that takes place through the transformations of consciousness. It is frictionless because it does not involve will or effort. Optimal health is preprogrammed into the nature of the human being to transform consciousness into matter and ultimately into the human experience.

The various levels of existence, the spiritual, mental, emotional, energetic and physical, are not merely concepts about separate states of being that exist when we simply ponder them. They are actual fields with different levels of vibrations, just as light waves are different from radio waves, but both are electromagnetic radiation.

For instance, as an irate supervisor yells, "I am not angry," she has tapped into two different levels of existence. She has part of her consciousness in the level of mental existence by voicing these words and at the same time, she has part of it in the level of emotional existence, which is characterized by her feelings of anger.

Dysfunction occurs when the levels are not integrated. When we say one thing and feel another, we become fragmented and disconnected, as these levels of our existence are no longer in agreement. Moreover, a whole and healthy life is created not just when the levels of our existence are in compatible communication with one another but when these levels are in contact with their source — consciousness.

## The Flow

Seven consciousness or energy transformers exist in the human physiology, each associated with different vibrations, functions and psychospiritual issues. Those who have studied Yoga know these as *Chakras*. Buddhist thought sometimes refers to them as the seven lotuses. They are described in terms of location, level of vibration of consciousness, psychology and physiology. On a physical level each relates to one of the endocrine organs in the body.

In Ayurveda they are called *Mahamarmas* or the great *Marmas*. Just like acupuncture points, they are responsible for the transformation of energy and consciousness into subtle flows through the channels or Srotas of the body.

The flow of consciousness starts at the absolute, where the frequency of vibration is so high it is immeasurable, hence the term absolute. It flows into the next levels all the way down until it reaches the physical level. Any blockage in its flow can create problems. Thus, disease can have its origins on different levels — spiritual, mental, emotional, energetic or physical. Knowing the level on which the blockage is occurring and how to rebalance it is one of the key components of Ayurvedic medicine.

Not every blockage is a psychological issue or a spiritual one. Put a poison in your body, and the problem is not on the psychological level. Positive thinking or resolving blockages to spiritual power cannot solve it.

The unbridled enthusiasm that accompanied the discovery of mind-body medicine led too many people to believe they could heal anything just by changing their minds. Ayurveda recognizes that disease can arise on many levels and that the wise healer addresses the root cause. This means addressing problems on the appropriate level.

## The Three Imperatives

This consciousness model gives us three imperatives, which are three keys to health. The first is that reconnecting with the source of health, the source of energy and intelligence, is vital to the process of healing.

The second imperative is that the smooth flow of consciousness and energy to the physical level must be maintained for health to be optimal. An obstruction on any level can hamper the flow of intelligence and energy necessary for natural healing. For instance, cancer can sometimes be due to a physical process, like pollution in the water supply, and sometimes it is due to emotional toxicity. Removing the toxins and the blockage before disease arises is considered the highest form of prevention.

The third imperative is that we must animate that which is life-giving and life-promoting. It originates in the principle that awareness can give life to anything. Just like watering a garden, we must attend to that which is in tune with our higher nature in order to create a healthy, productive, life-promoting lifestyle.

Since we have thus far concentrated on the theoretical concepts of health, we will now turn our focus back onto Charaka description of the purpose of Ayurveda and see how we know can understand that purpose.

# Charaka's Intention

Reconsider the Kaviratna translation (the more accurate one) of the purpose of Ayurveda according to Charaka:

> Mind, soul, and body, this trinity, called person, resteth on union like three sticks (standing with one another's support). Upon that (trinity) everything rests. That is also called *purusha* or being. It is also animate. That is regarded as the subject matter of this Science; and it is also for the sake of that, that this Science is promulgated.
>
> — *Charaka Samhita*
> *Kaviratna Translation*

With the understanding of the consciousness model, it is easy to put these words into context. We can see clearly the intention Charaka had. "Union" represents that underlying field of "being" that is indeed animate, since it is the source of all animate objects. (Remember each wave is made of water — water must be the essence of the ocean if the wave contains it.) This is the subject matter of Ayurveda. If we were to translate this in terms of the consciousness model in more modern language, we would translate Charaka as follows:

> **Mind, soul, and body, this trinity we call the human being, rests upon Unity (the unified field of consciousness); the whole world arises and is supported by this underlying Unity, just as a tripod is**

**supported by the ground beneath it. This unified field of consciousness, the Absolute transcendental reality, is called *purusha*. It is the source of life, animate and sentient. This is the true subject of this Veda we call Ayurveda. It is for the sake of knowing and experiencing Unity that this science is brought to light.**

Charaka understood that all the aims of life are undermined by ill health. He understood that the human being is involved in a process of growth and evolution — not in physical terms, rather in terms of knowing *all* of reality. Once the full reality dawns, once we know Unity, then we experience the field of consciousness and we know *how it works*. In this knowing, we can alter how it expresses itself in the patterns of balance or imbalance in the human physiology.

How does this relate to the science of Yoga? What is the purpose of Yoga? Popular notions would suggest its purpose is exercise. How does all of that relate to Ayurveda and its purpose?

# Yoga and Ayurveda

*Chapter 2*

# Yoga

Just as the esoteric knowledge of Ayurveda is fraught with confusion, so too is the understanding of Yoga. Just as the translators of Charaka were unclear about the structure of reality, so too, have many different versions and approaches evolved under the term "Yoga." Too often, Yoga is translated as "union of mind, body and spirit," as if its purpose is to adjust some fragmented parts of ourselves to work better together. This is, once again, the "tripod" without an understanding of what it rests on.

Yoga, as we will see, is "Union" — *union with the underlying field of consciousness itself.* To understand this fully, we need to understand the writings of the great yogis. Just as there were great sages who cognized the knowledge of Ayurveda, there were also those who knew the science of Yoga from their own experience of consciousness. The greatest of these sages was Patanjali.

Patanjali's Yoga Sutras make up the most concise, most profound, and probably most misunderstood set of writings that exist on the subject of Yoga. Just as the level at which Charaka was speaking was an evolved or enlightened one, so too with Patanjali. And, as with Charaka, he is subject to misinterpretation. Without a clear understanding of the consciousness model, and without a clear concept of how the evolution of consciousness occurs in the human being, we are lost in interpreting Patanjali.

The loss of the knowledge of consciousness and evolution has recurred throughout the ages. The common mistakes that undermine the continuation of the knowledge from generation to generation are easy to elucidate. When we come to know these common mistakes or errors in interpretation, we can see how the knowledge gets lost and how the different interpretations of Patanjali come about. We can, then, understand the confusion that exists in the realm of the practice of Yoga.

Two sets of concepts are required for us to even begin to approach Patanjali. The first is the common mistakes that are made in transmitting the knowledge of Yoga. The second set is an understanding of how consciousness develops in the human being. Both provide the context we need for understanding Patanjali and the purpose of Yoga.

## *The Loss of Knowledge*

Knowledge is lost when the student is not at the same level of consciousness as the teacher — a difficult situation when the subject matter is the development of consciousness itself. In this setting all forms of distortions can take place. We see this in the popular culture when some view Yoga as a religion. Certainly some practice Yoga religiously, but Yoga is not an Indian philosophy or religion. It is really about how the consciousness of all human beings works, regardless of creed or philosophy.

Yoga is not a "philosophy," rather it is a science of observation. Its principles are reproducible. Without an understanding of consciousness (i.e., without the consciousness model), the exposition gets turned into an intellectual distortion, a "philosophy," rather than a description of observations that are reproducible by any human being.

How did it come to be that this observational science is so misunderstood that it is thought of as a religion or a product of the Indian culture? How did it come to be that this practical application of techniques to develop consciousness has become so misunderstood?

### Householder and Monk

Part of the problem is that this knowledge has most recently been held in the ascetic or monk traditions of India. Thus, much of the tenor of Yoga, its practice and its interpretation has taken on the influences of ascetic practices of the monk tradition. What few people realize is that there is one path for the monk and a very different path for the householder.

The monk's path is based on loss and self-denial. The monk loses his family and society, loses all his or her possessions, gives up all control over the life and turns this over to the master. The monk undergoes ascetic practices and disciplines and loses more and more of his or herself until there is no ego or small "self" left. There is no attachment left to any part of the small self's life. Then dawns the experience of the larger Self, the transcendental reality. The wave becomes aware of the ocean beneath it and begins to experience it throughout the life. A state of nonattachment is achieved and eventually made permanent.

The householder's path is very different. It is not practical for the householder to give up family, society, money and possessions in the pursuit of evolving. It simply destroys both life and society to take this approach. The path of the householder is one of fulfillment. By becoming more and more fulfilled, by finding more and more fulfillment in midst of all activity, then the same state of transcendence is achieved and one becomes naturally nonattached.

To understand this, consider an analogy: Suppose a man is walking down the street and a pickpocket takes his wallet. What is the result? That depends on the inner state of the man. If the man is poor and homeless, the wallet may represent the very last money that he has, and its loss can mean that there will be no food to eat. The suffering and stress in this situation is tremendous. The man is very attached to the event and its impacts.

Suppose the same situation occurs: A pickpocket steals a man's wallet. But this time, suppose the man is a billionaire. What is the result? The billionaire has so much in the bank that it just doesn't really matter. He doesn't pretend it didn't happen, but it is only a minor nuisance for him — he just goes to the bank and gets more money and new credit cards and continues on his day. He is not attached to the event. It does not faze him. Why? Certainly not because he decides to pretend it didn't happen. It does not impact him because he *has so much.* When we are completely full inside — full of joy, fulfillment, and bliss — then we are naturally in a state of nonattachment. This is the path of the householder. It is one of heart, of bliss, of fulfillment of desires. The heart becomes so full of love and bliss that the events of life do not overshadow one's feeling of fulfillment. The householder's path is the path of bliss, and Yoga plays a central role in this path.\*

This is one of the key misunderstandings that plagues much of the Yoga literature and most of the translations of Patanjali. The result is all sorts of commentary about the suppression of desire and nonattachment, many of which make even the most repressive religions seem mild. Without a clear understanding of the different paths, we are lost. Serious students of Yoga will recall that there is a description of these two paths in the Vedic text known as the *Bhagavad-Gita*. In several chapters these two paths are described. In the 5th chapter, 2nd verse, the master explains to his student:

> Both renunciation and the Yoga of action,
> Lead to the supreme good, but of the two
> The Yoga of action is superior to the
> Renunciation of action.

The path of the householder is, in fact, faster than the path of the monk. In the words of the *Bhagavad-Gita*, it is "superior." Few people recognize this, for the path of the householder has been lost for so long. Thus, the knowledge of Yoga has

---

\* I am grateful to Maharishi Mahesh Yogi for this analogy.

been held in the ascetic traditions and too often it gets interpreted from that view. This is hardly what Patanjali or the other sages intended.

Yoga has nothing to do with suppressing desire or straining or stressing the body or with taking a religious or reverent view to life itself. These are remnants of the ascetic tradition that are neither appropriate for most of us, nor central to the core of what Yoga is.

## The End and the Means

The other very common mistake within the popular Yoga culture has to do with mistaking an end state for the path to that state. The Yoga master who is enlightened is the epitome of nonviolence and nonattachment. The student sees this and thinks this is the means: "If only I can act nonviolent and have loving compassion for all beings and be unattached to things, then I can make progress on my path." This illusion is propagated by those enlightened or near-enlightened individuals who do not remember clearly what it is to be unenlightened. For the enlightened, it is easy to remain unattached or to have loving compassion. But that is the result of their enlightenment. It is an analogous situation to "being in the moment." When a stressful event occurs, the enlightened will return to the peace and quiet of consciousness within them and the event will dissipate. They stay in the moment, and the stressful feelings dissolve. They don't get attached to the event or to the past memories and events that the situation might evoke. Thus, they don't suffer. So when their student is suffering, the teacher, having forgotten how it is to be unenlightened, reminds the student to just "be in the moment." Both teacher and student mistake this result of enlightenment — "being in the moment" — for the *means* to enlightenment.

This confusion is found everywhere in the Yoga literature. Nonattachment is the most common confusion. The enlightened are nonattached *because* of the state they have achieved, not because they have been "trying" to be nonattached. It happens spontaneously for them. It is the *result* of their inner state. We are attached until we are enlightened. To "try" to be nonattached is like playing the role of the president of the United States in hopes that if we do it well enough, we will become the president.

In the same vein of mistaking the end for the means, many books on Yoga say that the main principle of Yoga is *ahimsa* or nonviolence. And it is assumed that by "practicing" nonviolence we will attain to Yoga, to the state of enlightenment. This is like telling a child that if they practice standing on their toes they will grow to be tall as an adult. Nonviolence comes as a result of the growth of consciousness and the inner peace inherent therein. Nonviolence is not the *means* to developing consciousness.

Even the understanding of Yoga postures is fraught with this error. The ability to hold a posture with comfort for long stretches of time comes as a result of the development of consciousness, of awareness, as we will see in later chapters.

Nonattachment, being "in-the-moment," being imperturbable, having infinite flexibility ("going with the flow"), possessing infinite compassion — these are all the result of the development of enlightenment, the development of Union. These represent the end. When the means are not clear, and the student is not at the level of the teacher, then all sorts of distortions in knowledge and technique occur. Life is turned upside down and the end gets mistaken for the means.

**Description**
Patanjali's Yoga Sutras themselves represent this end-versus-means issue. What he was describing is indicated by Maharishi Sadashiva Isham (MSI) in the preface to his translation of the Sutras [*Enlightenement*, The Ishaya Foundation Publishing Company]:

Yoga is the Science of Union. The union of what with what? The union of the Waking State of Consciousness with its most expanded state. The fully developed state is called enlightenment. There are four stages of this development of higher consciousness; these are discussed in the four quarters of the Yoga Sutras.

Patanjali's Yoga Sutras are describing the higher states of consciousness, and not the means to them. It is like a satellite map — it provides all the detail of the terrain and it is very descriptive, but it doesn't tell you how to get from one point to the next. It is not a guidebook or a set of rules on how to travel a particular path. With all esoteric knowledge, one needs the context. Without the context, one does not have the key to unlock the truths that are contained within. Again MSI comments in his preface:

> The Yoga Sutras have been misinterpreted as the means to walk down the path to enlightenment. They are not. They are a description of the nature of enlightenment. Patanjali included no actual techniques of Ascension [transcendence] or Yoga in this text. His descriptions of the mechanics of enlightenment are so brilliant and clear, however, that many of the sutras have been widely misunderstood as actually being the techniques themselves.

The states that he describes, *and the organization of each state as one of the four quarters of the Sutras*, has been lost to many a generation. The descriptions of each of the four higher states of consciousness are descriptions of the end result — of the qualities of the experience — not the *means* to the experience.

The first quarter deals with the state of Transcendental Consciousness or Ascendance as MSI calls it. This is the direct experience of being, without thought, without sensory input — pure silence or pure consciousness as some might call it. The experience of being, of wakefulness without any input from the environment or the mind is what characterizes this state. The other names this state goes by are the Absolute, the Transcendent, pure awareness, and in Yogic terminology, Samadhi. These all refer to an experience of higher consciousness, one that differs from the states we are used to experiencing: waking, dreaming and deep sleep.

The second quarter deals with the higher state of consciousness known as Cosmic Consciousness or the state of No Mind, or Perpetual Consciousness. This is where the experience of Transcendental Consciousness has been fully integrated into the normal states of consciousness. That means that Transcendental Consciousness is experienced directly during waking, dreaming and deep sleep.

It sounds paradoxical without direct experience. Maintaining two states of consciousness is actually a well-documented capability of the higher mammals. Porpoises, for example, will sleep one half of the brain at a time. This is a necessity for them to be able to keep swimming and breathing. They are capable of functioning in two states of consciousness simultaneously. When the human nervous system continues to evolve and grow and integrate higher states of functioning and evolution with the normal states of waking, dreaming and deep sleep — then the human brain also maintains two states of consciousness simultaneously. The experience of Cosmic Consciousness is one of living the silence and experience of being or pure consciousness along with activity. All events have a quality of being "witnessed," as if one were watching them in a movie. Many musicians and athletes pop into this state briefly when they are "in the flow," "in the zone" or during a "peak experience." They describe the experience as silently watching it unfold perfectly and effortlessly. This is the witness aspect of this higher state of consciousness that comes from maintaining pure consciousness *with* activity.

The third quarter deals with the next higher state known as Glorified or God-consciousness. In this state, the subtle energies of creation start to be perceived along with the experience of silent being. Auras, energy fields, refined intuition and psychic phenomena are a standard part of the experience of this higher state. One begins to perceive the finer and more blissful aspects of creation. All of this gives the experience of life and the senses a glorified feeling, and a deep respect and love for all of creation (and the creator) tends to follow. Still at this stage there is a sense of the objects of perception being separate from the observer, although the energies that connect both may be perceived to be very connected.

The fourth quarter deals with Unity Consciousness. In this state, the perception of the subtle energies becomes so refined that there is a dawning of what lies underneath the subtle energies. That same, already-experienced silent being, experienced initially in Transcendental Consciousness and established in Cosmic Consciousness, is in fact the same thing out of which all of creation arises. When the experience of oneself — the silence within one's own being — is experienced as underlying all the subtle energies *and* all of what is observed, then there is a shift in consciousness and we realize that we *are* everything. We become the ocean and no longer just a wave on its surface. This is the state of Unity Consciousness, where reality has finally dawned and the illusion of the isolation of the wave dissolves.

What Patanjali is ultimately doing is painting the landscape of each of these states of consciousness. He is involved in giving us a description of the end. He is not providing the means, the methods or the techniques. When misinterpreted as the method, then Patanjali's "Eight Limbs of Yoga" get interpreted as steps to Yoga.

### The Eight Limbs

A common error in the translations of Patanjali's Sutras is that they are eight steps to Yoga and are they are commonly translated thus:

1. Yama (Restraints)
2. Niyama (Observances)
3. Asanas (Postures)
4. Pranayama (Breath Control)
5. Pratyahara (Sense Withdrawal)
6. Dharana (Concentration)
7. Dhyana (Meditation)
8. Samadhi (Absolute Bliss Consciousness)

Nowhere in the Sutras does Patanjali use the word "steps." There are no steps to Yoga, as is commonly interpreted. These are the limbs of a tree, all interconnected. They operate together. The fourth state of consciousness is the topic of the first quarter of Patanjali's Sutras. He does not introduce the limbs until the second quarter. What he is describing is how they are *affected by* the fourth state of consciousness as it becomes permanent or integrated into the other states of consciousness. He waits until the second quarter because he is describing a map of higher consciousness and elucidating the effects of Transcendental Consciousness on all the limbs of the life.

Life is an integrated whole. Patanjali was describing this whole, not the steps to it. It is like table with four legs. The table is an integrated whole, and when you pull one leg the entire table comes along. Patanjali is describing how these areas "come along" or develop as one experiences the fourth state of consciousness. What is that state? Samadhi — the main limb of the tree out of which the other limbs come and from which all the other limbs are nourished.

Becoming more flexible is a common experience of those practicing meditation techniques that create the experience of Samadhi. They carry less tension in the body and Asana practice becomes easier. Over time, the breath and breathing will tend to refine and become more efficient. One recovers from exertion faster than before — *Pranayama* or breath is affected and enhanced by the experience of Samadhi. Each limb is affected by the nourishment provided by the main limb (Samadhi).

Given this context and these keys, let us look at each of the eight limbs for a deeper understanding of the terrain that Patanjali is mapping out for us:

1. *Yama* — Translated as "to rein in, curb, bridle, discipline or restrain." Often these are described as the "restraints." The common misunderstanding is that these are the restraints or disciplines that are necessary in order to make progress on the path of Yoga — not so. Yama in the Vedic tradition represents death or the God of Death. Yama is therefore what we are dying to — what is departing us. The result is that negative habits are "reined in." But that is the result. What happens when the old bad habits die?

    a.  *Ahimsa* — Nonviolence
    b.  *Satya* — Truthfulness
    c.  *Asteya* — Non-stealing
    d.  *Brahmacharya* — Divine Conduct (*Brahma* = The Divine Creator *charya* = conduct or regimen)
    e.  *Aparigraha* — Nonattachment (literally "non-grasping")

Each day we experience the peace and silence of Samadhi we integrate this into our being and we naturally attain to nonviolence. We have more clarity and we recognize that lying always leads to problems in the end. We also see with this added clarity the impacts our actions have on others and therefore do not engage in harmful actions and do not engage in stealing. Our conduct becomes more divine and, as we have more experience of the bliss value of Samadhi, we are more full within ourselves and necessarily less attached. These five result from the experience of pure consciousness. They are the end, not the means.

2. *Niyama* — The prefix "ni-" negates what follows it in this Sanskrit language in the sense that it means "out" or "away from." So the opposite of or moving away from what we are "dying to" is that which we enliven or embrace. What is it that we enliven or embrace when we experience Samadhi or transcendence daily? Here is the list given by Patanjali:

    a.  *Shaucha* — purity

    b.  *Santosha* — contentment

    c.  *Tapas* — burning off of negativity ("tapasya" means heat)

    d.  *Svadhyaya* — self observance

    e.  *Ishvarapranidhana* — devotion to the Universal

Again, we see that as one practices meditation and experiences Samadhi, these are the results. Obvious to anyone is that such a practice will make for more purity and contentment and help us to release stress and negativity. And as we start to maintain some of the experience in our daily activity we will naturally be more self-aware and self-observant as we begin to experience the witness value of consciousness.

With the proper context we can understand what Patanjali was describing. Without it, Yoga becomes like a religion with a set of "do's" and "don'ts" — a continuation of a rather repressive approach to human development and spirituality. When we mistake the end that Patanjali is describing with the means to that end, we can create an ascetic, canonized set of guidelines that are an insult to life. We cannot live the fullness of life if we are forever thinking we are impure and must be disciplining ourselves with austerities.

3. *Asanas* — The word "asana" comes from the root "sa" or "stha" which means "to establish" or "to be established" in Sanskrit. It is the same root as *Sthapadya-Veda*, the science of

the natural laws of architecture. This is commonly translated as "postures." What is meant is to be established in the pose that one is taking. Patanjali clarifies this in another sutra using the word "asana" (one of three in the entire collection of Sutras). He states **Sthira sukham asanam**. Translated this phrase is composed of three words: s*thira* — stability or steadiness; *sukham* — sweet or pleasant; *asanam* — established pose or postures. When one is established, then the pose is steady pleasantness or stable sweetness. How does this relate to the development of consciousness? First, to be "established" is an often-used phrase in Vedic literature that refers to maintaining higher states of consciousness — it means to be established in that higher reality or heightened state of awareness. In that state, stress and tension are gone from the nervous system and the musculature. The posture is then naturally properly aligned, as no tension or old pattern or postural habit or memory pulls it out of its natural state of alignment. In that natural state, one is able to hold a posture without effort for long periods, up to hours, without fatigue and *with* a steady pleasantness — the sweetness of one's own bliss consciousness pervading the experience. Thus, once again, Patanjali gives us a description of the impact of higher consciousness on this "limb" of life — the result being steady pleasantness in posture or pose.

4. *Pranayama* — once again we see the word "yama." This time it references "prana" or breath. "Dying to the breath" or "the dying of the breath" is the more literal translation of this word. Unfortunately it has been translated as "restraint" or "control" of the breath and its original meaning has been entirely lost in methods of trying to restrain and control the breath. Patanjali in giving us a map of higher consciousness is alluding to the natural process that happens when we transcend. In the fourth state of consciousness the breath stops, often for 20-30 seconds or more. It literally "dies." Repeated exposure to this fourth state of consciousness results in refinement of the entire human physiology. It makes the breath more subtle and more shallow. Less deep and forceful breathing is needed to supply the body with

oxygen. This again results in a "dying of the breath" that is a predictable part of the development of higher consciousness. With this refinement all sorts of techniques and use of the subtle breath become possible. Again, the end, not the means, is what Patanjali describes.

5. *Pratyahara* — "Prati" means "away from"; "hara" means "food." Too often this is translated as restraining oneself from the pleasures of the material world, such as food. The deeper meaning here is in the word "food." What is the food that Patanjali is referring to? The Sutras thus far have had nothing to do with the daily existence or daily life. They have been focused on the internal experience — on consciousness and the workings of the mind. The mind contacts the world through the five senses. It finds fascination and interest outside of itself. The impression of the senses and the thoughts that arise as a result are the "food" of the mind. It is what feeds our interest and allows us to engage in the world. With the practice of meditation and the experience of Samadhi, we begin to experience the peace and then later the bliss of consciousness itself. The mind naturally "turns away" from its "food." This process of experiencing more bliss within oneself and turning within happens naturally as higher consciousness unfolds. Any attempt to "restrain" oneself from "pleasures" is trying to force the mind against itself — a process that is doomed to frustration and failure. It is confusing to life and it is a hindrance to living fully in the world in higher states of consciousness.

6. *Dharana* — The origin of this word comes from the Sanskrit "dhri" — "to hold." It is most often translated as "concentration" or "holding the mind in concentration." It is implied that this is a process, rather than a result. When something gains our fascination, the attention is held by it. It is this unwavering attention that comes with extreme fascination, not from a habit of forcing the mind to be still. What is the most fascinating, most blissful aspect in the state of higher consciousness? Pure consciousness itself is

described by the ancient sages as *sat chit ananda* — *sat* meaning "pure" — *chit* meaning consciousness — and *ananda* meaning "bliss." When the peace and silence of the settled mind that is attained in transcendental consciousness begins to deepen, the bliss value of consciousness begins to unfold. It is intensely blissful and can hold the mind in great fascination. When this begins to be carried over into the waking state of consciousness, the results are twofold. First, the ability to attend to things and find fascination in things grows. From an outsider's viewpoint, we appear to have greater powers of concentration. Second, the bliss of consciousness begins to be held simultaneously with all activity and all states of mind. It is like a white noise that is always in the background. Nothing is implied here by Patanjali about the means to enlightenment. He is describing the effect of the experience of Samadhi on the aspect of attention and its resultant ability to be held. Nowhere is there as much misunderstanding in the field of Yoga practice as in this particular limb. The insistence that concentration is the way to meditate and a necessary component of meditation is wholly misunderstood in the path of the householder. Concentration is the result of the settling of the mind, not the means to it. It is like a glass of water into which we have poured salt. As the salt settles to the bottom it becomes more concentrated. The "concentration" results from the *process of settling* that happens naturally, as opposed to us forcing the salt crystals to be compressed in some area of the water. Forcing the mind to "concentrate" is like making a project out of trying to force the crystals to be more compressed at the surface of the water. It goes against what is natural. It goes against the laws of nature that are working in that sphere. Effort and forcing are not the way for the householder.

7. *Dhyana* — Often translated as "to think" or "to meditate." When we misinterpret *Dharana* as the act of forcing the mind to concentrate, then the process of meditation also becomes misinterpreted. Thought in higher states of consciousness naturally leads one back to the transcendent. It is like a feather that falls off a bird. It naturally winds its way back to

the ground. Meditation for the householder is that process that will naturally lead the mind to the fourth state of consciousness, to the silence of pure consciousness. It occurs in a natural settling manner. As one begins to infuse the transcendental state of consciousness with the waking state, then the bliss of pure consciousness becomes more and more present. Thinking holds less fascination and will tend to trail back to silence and to pure bliss. Patanjali is describing that state of higher consciousness in which meditation is a natural component of moment-to-moment existence. He is describing how thought and meditation are infused with a different quality in the higher states of consciousness. Nothing in his Sutras implies effort, concentration or forcing of the mind.

8. *Samadhi* — From the root "sam" meaning "together" or "integrated" and the root "dha," which is similar to "dhri" meaning "to hold." Samadhi is that integrated state of consciousness where the union of mind and the underlying field of consciousness occurs. The two are "held together" and in that state, thought and sensation are transcended. It is the connection with the field of consciousness that creates the nourishment of all the other limbs. Why? Because pure consciousness is that field out of which all life and all liveliness arises. It enlivens every aspect of health and physical functioning, every aspect of cognition and mental functioning, and every aspect of the emotional life. It is the source of the sap that feeds all the other limbs. In higher states of consciousness, it is a living reality. Before that time, it is an experience that we have for moments until it is finally permanently integrated into the other states of consciousness.

\*\*\*\*\*\*\*\*\*\*\*\*\*\*\*\*\*\*\*\*\*\*\*\*\*\*\*\*\*\*\*\*

Without the knowledge of the path of the householder and the path of the monk — without the esoteric key about the four quarters and the states of consciousness they represent — it is easy to begin mistaking the end for the means. Like most esoteric books from the Vedas to the Bible, it is hard for us to understand them without the proper context and the proper keys.

Given these keys and the context of the consciousness model, what is Yoga and its purpose? Patanjali puts it very concisely:

### Yoga chitta vritta nirodhah

*Yoga* means "union" or to "yoke." *Chitta* is "consciousness." *Vritta* means "rolling" or "waves," and *nirodhah* means "elimination," "enclosed," "locked up" or "suppressed." Thus, Yoga is consciousness with the waves or vibrations of the mind eliminated. Unfortunately, many translators tend to use the word "suppressed." This gets into the problem of mistaking the state where the waves of thought are eliminated with the act of trying to suppress them. Patanjali is not talking about process. He is defining a state — what Yoga is.

When the thought-waves cease, then what has united with what? What is the Union? This is union of the individual being or individual consciousness with the unified field that underlies all of creation. It is the union of the individual self with the Universal Self. It is where the individual wave on the ocean experiences itself as the entire ocean. In modern language, then:

**Yoga is the union of the individual self with the unified field of consciousness, the Absolute transcendental reality that underlies all of creation.**

With this detailed and more accurate understanding of Yoga, we are prepared now to understand the relationship between Yoga and Ayurveda.

# Yoga and Ayurveda

*Chapter 3*

# Yoga & Ayurveda – Their Relationship

Let us look at the purpose of Ayurveda according to Charaka and the description and purpose of Yoga according to Patanjali.

According to Charaka, Ayurveda's purpose is described in modern terms as follows:

> **Mind, soul, and body, this trinity we call the human being, rests upon Unity (the unified field of consciousness); the whole world arises and is supported by this underlying unity, just as a tripod is supported by the ground beneath it. This unified field of consciousness, the Absolute transcendental reality, is called *purusha*. It is the source of life, animate and sentient. This is the true subject of this Veda we call Ayurveda. It is for the sake of knowing and experiencing Unity that this science is brought to light.**

According to Patanjali, Yoga is described in modern terms as follows:

> **Yoga is the union of the individual self with the unified field of consciousness, the Absolute transcendental reality that underlies all of creation.**

We see the sages are talking about one and the same thing. The subject of Ayurveda is for the sake of knowing and experiencing Yoga (Unity) — that is why Ayurveda exists. The great sages knew there was no greater impediment to growth and evolution than ill health. Ill health undermines all of life. In order to assure the individual continued growth and evolution toward greater awareness and greater bliss, they cognized the principles of health that are known as Ayurveda.

They also recognized this fundamental relationship: Health, growth, evolution and consciousness are not simply interrelated — they are essentially one and the same. Why? Because the source of life, the source of growth and evolution, comes from that same ocean of consciousness that underlies all of creation. Contact with that field enhances health; it enhances growth; it enhances evolution; and, it develops consciousness and individual awareness. Yoga, then, in its original sense, is fundamental to Ayurveda.

In reality, Yoga and Ayurveda are not sister sciences. They are an integrated whole. Yogic practices are an integral part of Ayurveda. Yoga is a modality of Ayurveda — perhaps the primary one. They were never meant to be separated. Just as the ancient physicians were also experts in astrology, the science of Ayurveda was never meant to be fragmented. This was the result of the loss of knowledge and of the systematic suppression of Ayurveda by the British that drove the knowledge of Ayurveda underground. In its resurgence, it has unfortunately taken on much of the fragmentation of the West, even to the point where many Ayurvedic schools in India are utilizing allopathic pharmaceuticals and shunning the practice of pulse diagnosis. Ayurveda has been misunderstood in the West as "Indian herbal medicine" that focuses on body types and nutrition. In fact, there are many modalities that are of greater importance in Ayurveda than nutrition and herbs. In order to understand that, we must understand how the human being works on many planes of existence simultaneously. We must understand how creation creates and how the different levels of the vibration of consciousness compose the different spheres of life — how we are essentially multi-dimensional human beings.

These spheres are known as the *Koshas* (literally "sheaths"). These are the sheaths that surround the individual consciousness and make up the spheres of existence that surround the experiencer — the mental, emotional, spiritual, energetic and physical spheres of human existence. Until the fourth state of consciousness becomes established, we tend to identify with one of these spheres (usually one more than another). We misperceive ourselves as our thoughts, or our feelings or the body. The unfortunate consequence of this misperception is the result of this fundamental truth — *any sheath can affect the others.* This means that our thoughts affect our physical body. This means that our beliefs affect our emotions. This means that our body affects our mood. It is all interrelated. To understand health means to understand the wholeness of the Koshas and their connection to the unified field. When we are healthy all of the Koshas are operating as an integrated whole and we have a strong connection to our source — to the underlying field of consciousness. Without this, we have a setup for disease and disaster.

One sheath can affect the other, because they are not separate. In fact, the dividing line between them is an arbitrary demarcation. At what point does a belief become more of a feeling? To understand the Koshas and how consciousness manifests itself as a physical body, we need to understand a little more about the consciousness model.

The underlying ocean of consciousness has no vibration. If we want to get technical and abstract, it has a vibration rate or frequency that is infinite. At the surface of the water, we have waves of various sizes and frequencies of vibration. It is the frequency of vibration that determines the level of existence or the Kosha that we are operating on. The spiritual level of life is a very high vibration, the mental level not as high, and the physical level is the lowest or densest of the vibratory levels.

Note that these vibrations are all occurring *in the ocean of consciousness.* They do not occur inside the individual. The concept that we are limited beings bounded by a bag of skin is one of the greatest illusions held by humankind. Each of these areas is a field that we tap into. At night, when we dream, for example, we are tapping into another field of existence, one with different laws of nature that can allow for us to walk through walls without thinking twice about it. We actually can meet others whom we know and can carry on conversations, although we usually don't remember much about the content. We can tap into the mental field and just "happen" to come up with the same idea that our friend proposes, or just happen to call our friend when they are picking up the phone to call us.

The human being, then, is an energetic system organized around different layers of consciousness. Each Kosha creates a layer in the energetic aura around the person, as a residual of our tapping into those fields. Ayurveda describes these layers as follows:

| Vedic Term | Analogous Concept |
| --- | --- |
| Annamaya Kosha | Physical Body / Physical Reality |
| Pranamaya Kosha | Etheric Body / Energetic Body / Physical—Nonphysical Interface |
| Manamaya Kosha | Astral Body / Emotional – Mental Reality |
| Gyanamaya Kosha (or Vijnanamaya) | Causal Body / Intuitive Reality |
| Anandamaya Kosha | Spiritual Body / Spiritual Reality |
| Atman | Higher Self / Transcendental Reality / Absolute Reality |

This understanding explains many healing phenomena that cannot be understood by a purely physical model. Distance healing, such as through prayer, is one example. Another example is psychic phenomena. In the consciousness model, vibrations of the unified field of consciousness are propagated like waves on an ocean. Anyone who develops the skill of tuning into subtle waves can get a sense of the vibrations of another person. This ability gives rise to psychic perceptions and psychic phenomena. Likewise, it gives us the ability to send vibrations and energy to another person in need of healing. Healing through prayer, or through "having one's aura adjusted" or through Healing Touch seems less farfetched when viewed through this model.

Furthermore, other psychic phenomena, such as knowing the future or knowing about other people without having met them, start to make sense. This sort of information can be obtained by raising one's awareness to the vibratory rate that corresponds with the intuitive level. At this level, information exists in symbolic form, the patterns of which give the template for creation and how it will unfold. Templates like these determine how the physical body will unfold. Just like this, other templates or forms give rise to the multiplicity of all creation. Those who can see these templates can see what might happen the future (assuming the template doesn't get altered).

In order to examine the relationship of Yoga, Yogic practice and Ayurveda in more detail, the Koshas need a little more explanation:

1. *Annamaya Kosha* — The Koshas or sheaths are sheaths of *maya*. Maya means "illusion." They obscure the reality and experience of the individual wave as being a part of the ocean. They are not "real" in the sense that they have no permanence. The waves come and go — it is the ocean that remains. *Anna* means "food." The physical body requires food and is composed of that solid level of life, just as is food.

2. *Pranamaya Kosha* — *Prana* means breath, but not in the physical sense, because this is not the physical level. It means the subtle energy that flows like the air we breathe, subtle and unseen. This is the energetic body — the area in which the acupuncture meridians and points exist (similar to the Marma points in Ayurveda). This is where the subtle channels or *nadis* exist and where the Pranic flows referenced in most of the Yoga literature exist. This is the level of the Chakras (see next chapter).

3. *Manomaya Kosha — Manas* means "mind." This is the level of the mind in Vedic terms. Mind in that system includes both emotion and the common or mundane thinking processes. Some esoteric systems make a division here between emotion and thought, and, therefore, have a seven-fold division. As mentioned, the map of the ocean of consciousness can be divided in different ways, because no line of demarcation exists between one level and the next. The Manomaya Kosha corresponds to the astral plane that we often experience at night in dreams.

4. *Gyanamaya Kosha* — This level is harder for most of us to understand because we have less direct experience of this until we undertake to develop our consciousness more. This is the intuitive level of life where many of the templates or subconscious patterns of the soul exist. It is called the "causal" plane in some esoteric writings. When the patterns that the soul is projecting into the life are enlivened with energy, they create habit patterns, lessons, tendencies, events, meetings and physical conditions. They *cause* the life to be organized in a certain manner, and, hence, this is called the *causal* level or plane of existence. When we tap into this level, whether it is in meditation, in a moment of clarity or in dreams, we can get an intuitive sense of the pattern, of what is to come. In fact, many of the creative solutions in science have come from tapping into this area of consciousness. Take the discovery of the structure of benzene (gasoline), for example. Chemists were puzzled for a long time about its structure. They knew it had six carbon atoms, but could not figure out how the bonds connecting them were arranged. Kekule, the chemist who solved this dilemma, had a dream of six snakes each biting the tail of the other, forming a ring. He awoke and knew immediately that the structure of benzene was a ring and not linear, like other hydrocarbons. *Gyana* means "intellect." This has

nothing to do with our concept of "intellectual." This level is high above the normal thinking of the mind that is in the Manomaya Kosha. It is the finest level of being able to discriminate and know "this" versus "that." It is very subtle. It is where we get a sense that something is right. It is almost beyond thought. At this level, intuition can be very lively. At this level, the causal patterns can be perceived. Short of that, there are important tools for getting a sense of the patterns with which an individual soul carries into this life. This is the utility of the system of Vedic astrology known as Jyotish. The Jyotish chart provides a glimpse of the patterns that exist on the causal plane in particular. The ancient Ayurvedic physicians were astrologers as well. Just as Yoga was never meant to be separated out from Ayurveda, neither was Jyotish. Jyotish is important, not only in being able to perceive the causal patterns, but in providing important remedies for altering the patterns and countering the energies that are coming forth into the life from this plane of existence. When Ayurveda is studied without Jyotish, a fifth of the multi-dimensional human being is lost.

5. *Anandamaya Kosha — Ananda* means "bliss." The highest realms of consciousness carry with them more of the essential nature of consciousness, which is bliss. This is the realm of the angels, guides and archangels described in much of the esoteric literature. Here information is highly symbolic and highly organized. The senses tend to be merged and sounds create visual forms. The highest vibration brings with it the joy and ecstasy that inspire the mystical poets and writers. This is the region that many have caught glimpses of using hallucinogenics (and hence the draw to these drugs). The problem with these drugs is that throwing the nervous system into this realm before it is ready can damage it. In addition, drugs can't give you permanent access the way developing consciousness can. (Hallucinogens are

like shifting from first gear to fourth gear in an expensive Lamborghini — you are likely to leave your transmission on the pavement behind you.)

Ayurveda is practical knowledge. Thus far we have been laying the groundwork for understanding the practical application of Yoga and Ayurveda. The Koshas give an important understanding for the practice of Ayurveda, if we understand how health is created and Yoga's rightful role in that process. Suppose we want to create the perfect heart. The template for this is not just in the DNA — that's why scientist can't figure out how a single cell (the ovum) "knows" how to divide and make the different parts of the fetus. Here is a simple, although somewhat crude way to understand the Koshas and the unfolding of the perfect heart:

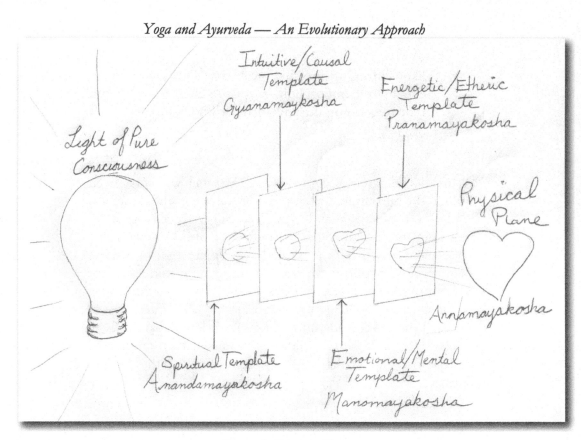

Diagram by Kristen Spalding

To create the perfect heart, we have to have the light of pure consciousness pass through the template that exists in each Kosha. Any distortion or problem or weakness in the light will lead to problems on the physical level. For example, a distortion on the level of the emotional template (a lonely, broken heart) can affect the physical heart. This is being increasingly recognized even in allopathic medicine, where the work of Dr. Dean Ornish has shown that one of the commonalities in heart disease patients is an underlying isolation or loneliness, even if they married. Ornish saw this effect so consistently that he began requiring counseling for all his heart patients.

If we understand this refinement of the consciousness model, we can see that with Ayurveda we have an understanding of how consciousness, spirit, mind, emotions, energy and the body are interrelated. This brings us both great understanding and great power.

First, it brings us the power to precisely diagnose the level from which a problem originates. Some problems are physical. If you ingest some contaminated scallops and get food poisoning, it doesn't matter how many affirmations or Yoga postures you do. If you take the wrong diet for 20 years, you may end up with a physical problem from a physical cause. However, the vast majority of health problems do not originate at the physical level. Even the allopathic physicians know that the majority of the problems they see are related to stress, to emotional habits (such as emotional eating), to addictions and to beliefs that get in the way of maintaining health. Ayurveda has the power to discriminate the level at which these originate and the means for accurately diagnosing these.

Second, and more important, Ayurveda has tools for intervening on each level. This why Yoga, Jyotish and meditation cannot be separated out of Ayurveda. The attempts to make Ayurveda an herbal version of modern medicine betray its essence as a comprehensive holistic system of knowledge — one that understands all the levels of creation and human existence. It understands all of nature and how nature unfolds. The power to intervene on these other levels is central to its efficacy. It gives rise to the many modalities that are a part of Ayurveda. Here are some examples from the subtlest to grossest:

1. *Anandamaya Kosha (Spiritual Level)* — If the problem is arising from this level — say a spiritual disconnection or isolation is creating a depression, then one technique available to the Ayurvedic physician is meditation. Meditation allows one to reconnect with the greater whole and allows one to contact the "ananda" value or the bliss value of consciousness. It is a powerful tool if the depression is arising from this level.

2. *Gyanamaya Kosha (Causal Level)* — If a problem or condition, such as depression, is arising from a subconscious pattern, it may be one that was brought with the soul into this life or what is called a "Karmic" pattern. If it is, then, this can be seen in the Jyotish chart. There are many Jyotish remedies for dealing with problems on this level, for altering Karma. The use of gemstones, the use of symbolic patterns called *Yantras*, the use of *Yagyas* or vibrations that are sent into the unified field to alter the vibrations coming to an individual — these are all examples of the types of modalities that can be used to correct problems originating from this level.

3. *Manomaya Kosha (Mental/Emotional Level)* — Most of the problems confronting individuals in the developed nations arise from this level. Aromatherapy is a powerful modality for assisting on this level. The human brain is wired with direct connects from smell to the limbic system or the emotional brain. Meditation is also powerful on this level, bringing awareness to our subconscious patterns and destructive patterns, so that we can change them. Music or sound therapy, called *Ghandharva-Veda* is another powerful modality on this level. There are many consciousness-based techniques for operating on this level, ranging from the utilization of subtle mantras to specific Yogic practices to clearing emotional patterns, traumas and cellular memories (see Chapter 6).

4. *Pranamaya Kosha (Energetic or Etheric Level)* — This is the level where the techniques of Yoga operate most fully and effectively. Being able to re-establish energetic flow and to clear and enliven the energy centers in the body (the Chakras) is the forte of this modality. Elizabeth Haich describes the power of these techniques in her book *Initiation* [Aurora Press, 2000] where she describes having also utilized these techniques in a past life in Egypt: "Every morning at

sunrise we have to assemble in the garden. We begin with physical exercises… We assume various body postures and, while doing breathing exercises, must guide our consciousness into different parts of the body. Through long and patient practice in this way we can make the entire body completely conscious, move at will, control and guide the smallest parts of the body and all internal organs. Patiently and persistently we thus develop the body into an excellent instrument." Ayurveda also uses the acupuncture meridian system. "Marma" points or Marma Therapy, or stimulation of Marma points is a powerful modality of intervention on this level.

5. *Annamaya Kosha (Physical Level)* — Physical techniques from massage, to purification therapies (*Panchakarma*), to diet, to herbs, to Vedic architecture (*Sthapatya-Veda*) operate on this level. Certainly these all can operate on more subtle levels as well. Herbs do have a higher vibrational aspect that influences mind and emotion. Their effect, though, is more physical in nature. Diet also plays a huge role in emotion and food can be a carrier for emotional, spiritual and subtle energies. However, it has a huge impact on the balance of the physical level of life, and the Ayurvedic understanding of this impact goes far beyond that seen in other systems of medicine.

Finally, and most important, this understanding of the human being allows us to detect imbalances long before disease arises. This is medicine taken to its supreme form. Detecting an imbalance on the mental or causal level *before* it has had a chance to affect the physical body is an invaluable part of this medical science. It is consistent with Patanjali when he says in his Yoga Sutras:

### Heyam dukta anagathum
"Avert the danger not yet come."

Ayurveda in ancient times was mainly preventive in its nature. The physicians were only paid if the village was healthy. The value of a truly preventive system of medicine in modern times cannot be overstated. Understanding the Koshas and how consciousness works gives us the keys to intervene long before disease arises. We can truly avert the danger before it comes.

The relationship between Yoga and Ayurveda becomes clear with the understanding of the Koshas. Yoga and Ayurveda were never meant to be separated into different bodies of knowledge. They are one and the same. Yogic practice is a valuable part of Ayurveda, particularly for working on the level of the Pranamaya Kosha. Furthermore, the goal of Yoga cannot be reached without utilizing the subtle techniques of Ayurveda.

Yoga, Jyotish, Sthapatya-Veda — all cannot be separated from Ayurveda. Any attempt to do so demonstrates a lack of understanding of Charaka and Patanjali and the essential nature of what Ayurveda is. We cannot divide the human being into pieces and parts and hope for health. Ayurveda stands for wholeness. It is complete in its understanding and practice. And Yoga is an integral part of that whole.

# Yoga and Ayurveda

*Chapter 4*

OJAS & AMA, PRANA & CHAKRA

# Ojas & Ama, Prana & Chakra

Our ability to live, to love, to create and prosper in the world all depend on the physical body. Consciousness drives the manifestation of the body and the body's health is dependent on the health of the connection with the underlying field on consciousness. In creating health, the first imperative is that the connection to our liveliness, to our source, be strong. Without this, balance or imbalance, proper diet or improper diet, right routine or no routine at all — everything else is inconsequential.

Once again the importance of meditation and of contacting the underlying field is of paramount utility in creating health. Just as Samadhi nourishes all the limbs of Yoga, it actually is the one technique that enlivens all of the Koshas. It must be put at the forefront of both Yoga and Ayurveda in considering health.

Ayurveda goes deeper in its understanding of how this contact works — what is required, how it can be enhanced, and how it feeds the Prana and Chakra systems described in Yogic literature. The contact of the physical with the nonphysical is mediated through a very refined substance called Ojas.

Ojas is thought to be the byproduct of perfect digestion and is said to exist on the physical level and have physical qualities. Yet, its functions are nonphysical. It is like a wire that can conduct electricity — no attempt to dissect the wire will allow one to see how it functions in carrying electrical current. Ojas is perhaps more similar to a crystal in its interaction with the nonphysical aspects of the human being. In the beginning days of radio, a small crystal was used that would vibrate when certain frequencies of electromagnetic energy (radio waves) would hit it. The crystal would take the radio waves and transform them into electricity that was vibrating in sync with the pattern of the radio waves. In this manner the nonphysical was turned into current that could physically move a speaker and produce sound.

Ojas is like a crystal. It transduces the "waves" of consciousness into "life force." It is responsible for much of our liveliness and physical energy. Interestingly enough, the more consciousness we imbibe into the physical, the more Ojas increases (it works both ways). According to Sushruta, the great Ayurvedic surgeon, Ojas is that which nourishes every part of the body. Why? Because the liveliness and the health of the body is dependent on its contact with the underlying field of consciousness, and Ojas is responsible for that contact. Ojas is also responsible for strength and immunity. Here is what Sushruta said about Ojas:

> The pure intelligence or essence of the Dhatus [tissues] is called auspicious Ojas and also Bala [strength, immunity]. By Bala or Ojas, Mamsa [muscle tissue] becomes full, all movements become free and perfectly coordinated, voice and complexion become clear, and externally and internally the activity of the organs of action and the sense organs become Self-referral [connected with consciousness], intelligent and evolutionary.

> Ojas, which is of the nature of soma [the plant kingdom's interface with consciousness], is: unctuous, white, cool, stable, moving, flowing, pure, soft and cohesive. And is located at the very sprouting of life, of Prana. Being omnipresent in living beings, Ojas nourishes every part of the body. Deficiency of Ojas is equal to the destruction of the body of living beings.
> — *Sushruta Samhita (15. 19-22)*

Ojas and its creation become crucial to all of life. To focus on balance (Doshas) or on tissues (Dhatus) before focusing on Ojas puts the cart before the horse. Dosha balance means nothing if there is no Ojas, for as Sushruta points out, lack of Ojas is equal to the destruction of the body.

Note also that Ojas is present at the sprouting of life. Prana, or the subtle energies of the body, is dependent on Ojas as well. Ojas is like a lamp near a doorway. It shines both in the room in which it is located and in the room to which the doorway leads. Ojas's "room" is the physical body and the room it shines into is the Pranamaya Kosha — the subtle energy body or etheric body, as it is called in the esoteric literature.

Unfortunately, the term "Prana" gets thrown around a lot in modern writings on Yoga and sometimes is equated with consciousness itself. In some writings, different types of Prana are even discussed. This confusion comes without a deep understanding of consciousness and the composition of the Koshas. Prana is that vibration of consciousness operating near the interface between the physical and nonphysical aspects of the human. It makes up the "Chi" that flows through the acupuncture meridians and the *nadis* or subtle channels in the Ayurvedic system. It is responsible for the liveliness, flow and warmth of the body.

Prana, then, as every Yoga practitioner needs to know, is dependent on Ojas. What enhances Ojas? What will decrease it? A modern translation of Charaka's opinion on factors that increase Ojas yields the following:

1. *Good digestion and balanced diet:*
   Ojas is the end product of a whole series of transformations that occur when metabolizing food. Enhancing our ability to assimilate and transform food increases the possibility that we will end up with more Ojas being formed in the digestion process.

Note that this comes even before balanced diet in its importance. Obviously, without the proper components body tissues and Ojas itself cannot be formed, so balanced diet is important.

2. *Love, joy, and appreciation — positivity in feelings, speech and behavior:*
   Although Ojas is a physical substance, it is affected by nonphysical events. Just as the entire body is affected by the templates in the layers of consciousness above it, so too, the body's production of Ojas is directly enhanced by love and appreciation. This concept ties in well with the current findings in mind-body medicine that show enhanced immunity when love is experienced in life. Immunity is the modern term for an increase in strength (Bala) that comes with increased Ojas.

3. *Panchakarma:*
   These are the Ayurvedic purification therapies that remove impurities from the body and are said to improve the cells' ability to wake up and receive Ojas.

4. *Rasayanas:*
   These are special Ayurvedic herbal and mineral substances that are potent tonics or rejuvenators of the physical body. The classical formula *Chyavanprash* is based on the most rejuvenative herb in the Ayurvedic pharmacopeia (Amalaki) and is perhaps the most well-known Rasayana in modern times. It is the basis for the *Amrit Kalash* formula.

5. *Consciousness:*
   Last but not least, developing consciousness also "upregulates" Ojas in the body and makes it more available. In this manner, more energy and liveliness are able to be conducted to the physical body itself.

In practical terms, Ojas appears in the healthy as the glow of the skin, the twinkle or pleasant wateriness of the eyes, in the pleasantness of the voice and the vibrancy of energy that such a person exudes. Any student of Yoga who wants to develop the ability to practice Asana needs to be aware of how to enhance Ojas, because Prana is dependent upon it. They also need to be aware of factors that Charaka and other Ayurvedic sages noted as responsible for decreasing Ojas. These include:

1. *Hurrying or entertaining negative emotions, (i.e., stress):*
   Stress is known to be a major factor in the cause of disease. It is perhaps the greatest factor in developed nations. Hurrying is usually a result of worrying or stress and is probably related in this fashion. The stress of negative emotions is also significant. Note, however, that nothing here indicates suppression of negative emotions. There is no prescription against having them. We don't make a mood of not having negative emotions. That only creates further stress. The key word here is "entertaining." Once a negative emotion comes up we don't invite it to remain and come to dinner and sit with us through the evening. We let it go, rather than reinforcing it.

2. *Excessive exercise:*
   Exercising too much depletes the life force and Ojas. It makes one age faster. Look at the skin and faces of marathon runners. You can see the depletion of Ojas and see the aging process accelerating. Correct exercise is very useful. It improves our ability to digest food and actually enhances Ojas. The question becomes one of what is "excessive"? Weakness after working out is a sign of reduction of Ojas. We should feel enlivened by exercise, not exhausted.

3. *Fasting excessively:*
   In general, fasting is not favored in Ayurveda for this reason. Occasionally fasting for a day is not so

damaging to Ojas. But any more than this is considered excessive and will take away from the life force.

4. *Rough or very light diet:*
This reality doesn't fit so well with what many people conceive of as a healthy diet. The problem with the meat-based diet of the modern American culture is that it is devoid of fiber, fruits and vegetables. Emphasizing more fresh foods has become quite popular. In fact, the trend in many health-conscious people has swung to the other extreme and to "go raw." The problem with a raw-foods diet was seen by the ancient Ayurvedic sages. A rough diet, or a diet that is too light, will aggravate the balance of the body (*Vata Dosha*) and weaken the digestive fire (assimilation and metabolism) over time. Ultimately, the weakness in digestion results in the production of less Ojas. This is not just a theory in applying Ayurveda to modern times. It was observed by the ancients long ago.

5. *Overexposure to wind and sun:*
Sunburn and windburn leave one exhausted. It is the Ojas-depleting effect of these events that can zap the life force and leave one tired.

6. *Staying awake through much of the night (sleep deprivation):*
No other area of life is taken for granted as much as is sleep. Charaka knew the impact of sleep deprivation on Ojas and advised that sleep be regarded as important as diet. He described how all of life depends on proper sleep. In modern society, sleep deprivation represents one of the main Ojas-depleting factors.

7. *Dehydration or excessive loss of body fluids (blood):*
Blood and water nourish the entire physiology. You cannot sustain life if you lose too much of either.

8. *Overindulgence in sexual activity:*
   This is not a prescription for avoiding sex and for repression of sexual desire. Just as excessive exercise can deplete the life force, so too can excessive sexual activity. Just as proper exercise can enhance Ojas, so too can proper sexual activity enhance Ojas (as it enhances love). The key is to know what "excessive" means. Just as with exercise, this is an individual consideration. If one feels exhausted, moody, depleted after sexual activity, then that is a sign that it has probably been excessive. Again, one should feel enlivened, more awake, more aware and more loving after sexual activity.

9. *Injury or trauma to the body (including surgery):*
   There is a "shock" effect to trauma or surgery that depletes the body's energy. It is a physical stress reaction as opposed to an emotional one. This stress decreases the life force and leaves one exhausted after trauma.

10. *Alcoholic beverages:*
    Once again, modern culture could well learn from the ancient sages in this regard. It was not a judgment the sages made of "good" versus "bad" when it came to alcohol. They were simply stating the known effects. Alcohol is very Ojas depleting. It is, in essence, a poison or a toxin that the body must work to clear. It is known in Western science to be a potent producer of free radicals that can damage all aspects of the human physiology. This decreases the life force.

Understanding Ojas is crucial to health. It is more fundamental than balance or toxin buildup because without it, there is no life force and eventually no life at all. Loss of Ojas is at the root of many patterns of ill health — the particular imbalance that manifests with the ill health is just an interesting footnote, not the essential story.

By promoting Ojas we promote Prana and the flow of subtle energy in the body. This flow is important to health, to spiritual development and the development of consciousness. While Prana flows in subtle channels throughout the body, there are two main conduits that are well-described in the Yogic literature. These spiral up from the base of the spine around the spinal column up to the head. These subtle energy channels are called *Ida* and *Pingala*:

> **Pingala** is associated with solar energy, positive polarity and masculine or outgoing energy. The word *pingala* means "tawny" in Sanskrit. Pingala has a sunlike nature and male energy. Its temperature is heating and it courses from the left groin to the right nostril. Pingala is the extroverted, solar Nadi, and corresponds to the left-hand side of the brain.

*[handwritten margin note: Wheating / L Brain / R. Nostril / Male]*

> **Ida** is associated with lunar energy negative polarity and female or receptive energy. The word *ida* means "comfort" in Sanskrit. Ida has a moonlike nature and female energy with a cooling effect. It courses from the right groin to the left nostril. Ida is the introverted, lunar Nadi, and refers to the right-hand side of the brain.

*[handwritten margin note: Female / Cooling / L Nostril / R Brain]*

These two spiral up the spine and where they intersect form the Chakras (literally "wheels"). At the intersection the two diverse currents causes a spinning effect that creates the energies of the Chakras. When these two spiral up properly, then the rest of the Pranic flows in the body tend to be nourished and flowing properly as well. The result is vibrant health. This is not something that is just a theory of Indian culture. The knowledge of the Chakra system and these Pranic flows is well-known in esoteric literature and in the mystical traditions of most of the world's religions. It was understood by the Greek physicians, for example. Few people realize that the symbol for the medical profession (the caduceus) is referring to these channels and that health is created when there is proper flow. Here is an illustration of the caduceus:

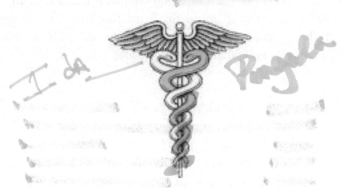

The Pranic flow of Ida and Pingala are represented as snakes that wind their way up a staff. In this representation the Chakras are omitted, and the staff is utilized to represent the spine. Once again we see that the knowledge of Yoga is intimate to the knowledge of health.

With the knowledge of Ida and Pingala we also gain knowledge of the origins of a popular term "Hatha Yoga." *Ha* means "sun" and *tha* means "moon." So this form of Yoga unites the energies of the sun (Pingala) and moon (Ida). Sometimes "Hatha" is translated as "to force" when in fact it mostly likely refers to the noun "force" that is the force or energy of Ida and Pingala.

When the two channels intersect they form the Chakras. These relate to specific energies and functions in the mind-body system. While they are primarily the Pranic flows on the Pranamaya Kosha, they have higher vibrations or "overtones," as it were, that impact the other Koshas, particularly the emotional/mental level or Manomaya Kosha.

There are seven Chakras in total. Each one is associated with an area of the body, with the endocrine system to be more precise. Each one relates to psychospiritual issues, and each one is more than just a flow of "energy." Remember that consciousness, that sea out of which all of the Koshas arise, is more than just energy. It is intelligence or organizing power. It carries both energy and information and is creative in its focus. What is created with each Chakra is a re-enlivenment of patterns of energy, belief and emotion. The Chakra system gives a window into the organization of the egoic structures as well. These obviously are restructured as the individual evolves toward higher states of consciousness. Even though they are created by the flows of Prana through the etheric plane, their higher harmonics produce impacts on the emotional and mental planes.

The Chakras also have correspondences with the planets in the Jyotish system. The causal energies (the higher vibrations) often influence the functioning of the Chakras. Here is an overview of the Chakra system, first from the standpoint of function:

# Chakras

| Chakra | Name | Major Function |
|--------|------|----------------|
| 1 | Muladhara (Root) | **Physical Identity – Security and sense of belonging.** Stores our experience and memories of family / community (tribe) – our cultural heritage and upbringing and our sense of belonging in a community. **Self-Identity** |
| 2 | Swadhisthana (Sweetness) | **Emotional Identity – Emotions, the feeling sense and one-on-one relationships.** Stores our memories and experiences in close relationships of all kinds, including sexual experiences. **Self-Gratification** |
| 3 | Manipura (Lustrous Gem) | **Ego Identity – Self-esteem and sense of autonomy.** Stores our memories and experiences related to our independence, our ability to achieve in the world, and our sense of personal competence or power. **Self-Definition** |
| 4 | Anahata (Unstruck) | **Social Identity – Benevolent and Divine Love.** Stores our memories of love and of our connection to the Divine. **Self-Acceptance** |
| 5 | Vissudha (Purification) | **Creative Identity – Will to create and to express.** Stores our memories and experience with speaking up and speaking out, with our creativity and our will to create. **Self-Expression** |
| 6 | Ajna (To Perceive and Command) | **Archetypal Identity – Ability to perceive.** Stores our patterns of perception and our intuition – our ability to know on a subtle level and to perceive the archetypal pattern we are manifesting. **Self-Reflection** |
| 7 | Sahasrara (Thousand-Fold) | **Universal Identity – Connection with the Divine Truth.** Houses our connection to Spirit and to Universal Truth. **Self-Knowledge** |

In order to understand the Chakras we must understand that they store impressions, emotions and memories, as well as serving as a source of energy. In order to understand this patterning, we need to draw on the concept of "cellular memory." Most of us have the illusion that memory is stored in the brain. The experience of transplant patients would argue against this concept. Memory can occur on the cellular level and the memory imprints on one organ can get passed to another individual in the transplant process.

One of the clearest examples of this was the story of a transplant patient in her late 40s. She had been born with a defective heart, and she knew that she had to take care of herself if she did not want to die at a young age. Even with optimal self-care, she knew that she would require a heart transplant at some point in her life. She was very fastidious about diet and became a vegetarian at a young age and had not eaten any meat in many years when she received her heart transplant. Shortly thereafter, when she left the hospital, she noticed that she started to have cravings for meat. What was also strange was that her cravings were very specific — she kept having the desire for a McDonald's hamburger. She started noticing all the McDonald's restaurants as she drove around the city. This was so uncharacteristic, and the timing so close to receiving her new heart, that she began to wonder if there was any connection. She obtained permission to contact the donor's family and learn more about him.

She discovered that he was a 19-year-old man who had just moved away from his parents at age 18. He did not know how to cook. Even before moving from his parents' home, his favorite restaurant was McDonald's, and after he lived on his own, he ate there almost every day. She began to talk with transplant researchers about this phenomenon, as it appeared that she was having memories and cravings that were coming from her new heart and not from her personality.

Her story is one that illustrates dramatically the reality that cells are more than just collections of cellular "parts." It shows that impressions and subtle energies are stored in the body — that the memory of events, traumas and emotions get stored in the body at a cellular level. The human "nervous" system is not where memory is stored. It is actually located diversely in subtle fields throughout the body — it is really a system of consciousness. The vibrations of consciousness permeate the physical body just as a wave will ripple across a whole pond.

The Chakras are part of this energetic system of memory and experience. The Chakras are associated with the endocrine system. The endocrine system is composed of "ductless" glands that work by emitting biochemical messenger molecules that affect the entire body. The adrenal gland, for example, releases adrenalin that causes the heart to race, the blood pressure to elevate, the pupils to dilate, the hairs of the skin to "stand on end" and blood sugar to elevate. These messenger molecules affect the body as a whole. The Chakras are associated with these glands and hence have widespread influence on the physical body and on health. But the Chakras also have energetic, emotional and mental effects as well. They store information. Perhaps a more accurate way of thinking of them is as energetic information databases that can be read and understood by those sensitive to the subtler vibrations of consciousness.

Typically the types of information and functions stored in the Chakras are similar between human beings. Just as the effects of the adrenal hormones are predictably different from those of thyroid hormone, the types of information and emotional issues vary from Chakra to Chakra. In this manner, we have a system of energetics that can be described with typical patterns and characteristics.

**Chakras 1 – 3: The Egoic System**

The first three Chakras have to do with what would be called the ego in both modern psychological terms and in esoteric terms. One's identity or one's limited sense of self is related to the functions of the first three Chakras. The ego structures result in a sense that we are separate, isolated, with a personality uniquely ours. This limited sense of self is very different from the broad sense of self we experience in higher states of consciousness.

When one is under the illusion of the ego, life is very scary. As an isolated being, there is loneliness. As identified with the body, we can die at any moment. The life of the ego-bound person is one of fear. All of the structures of the ego are organized around managing survival and the resultant fear of destruction. For example, if I believe that by being different I risk being ostracized from my society, then I will do anything to conform — if I don't, I won't be able to survive. Standing up in front of a group of people to give a speech in this setting becomes a terrifying event. "What if they don't like what I have to say?" "What if I forget my speech?" "What if I get booed off the stage?" The ego perceives these events as leading to ostracism and demise. Perhaps from our ancient heritage, where being ostracized from the tribe *did* mean that we would be die, we carry in the subconscious mind the memory of past trauma that does evoke the fear of ostracism — thus making giving a speech a life-and-death situation for many.

The first three Chakras are all organized around the ego and its prime dictate of survival. To understand the first three Chakras, we need only ask, "What does this Chakra have to do with survival?" Analyzed from this viewpoint, the first Chakras are as follows:

1.  *Chakra 1: What group do I need to belong to or what do I need physically in order to survive?*
    The 1st Chakra is related to security. It is our physical base. What do we need physically in order to feel secure? For some, this can be a physical space, a big

61

house or big bankbook. For the vast majority, however, through lifetimes of conditioning we have taken as our security the tribe we belong to. In our human history, survival has depended on our ability to be part of the group, part of the society. In that ancient ancestry, we became conditioned to associate being thrown out of the tribe with a fate worse than death. This conditioning places our security in the hands of the tribe. For most of us, then, fitting into a family, a peer group or a social circle is paramount to survival. Whatever issues we have related to survival and security get stored in this Chakra and alter its functioning. It relates to the structures we create for security, both physically and mentally. As we evolve, the security we seek comes in a different form. With the experience of higher consciousness, we come to understand that the body may perish, but we continue on. We begin to see that our survival is not dependent on others, but on our own Karma and on the Universal and our attunement with that. The enlightened 1$^{st}$ Chakra does not need to look outside for security and with this flow of higher vibration, the grip of the impressions that reside in this Chakra no longer hold power over the person or their experience.

2. *Chakra 2: What close relationships do I need in order to survive?*

The 2nd Chakra is mainly about emotion. It is all about the emotions and the emotional connections that we have needed in order to survive. It is also about the bliss that comes when the emotions flow. Unfortunately, because sexual relationships also play out in this Chakra, the common association of this Chakra in popular literature is with sex and sensuality. In fact, the impressions and psychological programming that often reside here have as much to do with our parents as with our lovers. Remember, the ego perceives that it is necessary to our survival to have these relationships. For most of our childhood, we reinforced the notion that we needed our parents in order to survive, even if they were abusive and destructive to our survival. These emotional patterns often get played out in our friendships, in our romantic relationships and often with our own children. Most of our feelings of need, of dependency, of being loved and all that we do in order to have this kind of love — all of these patterns and emotions — are stored in the 2nd Chakra. All kinds of addictions and dependencies are stored here. Sexual experience and the ability to experience sensual pleasure in all its forms are also a part of the 2nd Chakra. In "all its forms" refers to the ability to appreciate art and beauty, luxury, opulence and wealth. The 2nd Chakra is intimately related to our bankbooks. The ability to flow abundant wealth is an expression of the flow of energies through the 2nd Chakra. Dealing with emotion, wealth, abundance and sexual relationships, the 2nd Chakra plays a huge part in the human life. With the development of higher consciousness, the dependency and destructive emotional patterns tend to fade away. The bliss of pure consciousness provides an inner means to happiness that takes the draw away from addictions. The enlightened 2nd Chakra allows one to enjoy the flow of abundance and sensuality without an addiction to them. Emotional clarity comes and great bliss dawns in all arenas of life.

3. *Chakra 3: What do I need to accomplish and what personal power do I need to demonstrate in the world in order to survive?* The 3rd Chakra is all about autonomy and self-esteem. If we perceive ourselves as inadequate, lacking in worth, and ineffective, we become shy, insecure and don't trust ourselves in the world. For some these feelings are suppressed, and they engage in over-compensation. The overachiever, the "Type A" personality, the braggart and the bully are usually trying to avoid their insecurities and prove that they are fully functional and powerful in the world. The

3rd Chakra is about what we need to accomplish in the world, what work we need to do in order to feel autonomous and independent. It brings with it the sense of personal effectiveness. The enlightened 3rd Chakra carries with it an awareness of the support of the Universal in all endeavors. It knows its worth is not dependent on accomplishment; rather that it is inherent in being. Survival, self-worth and accomplishment are not dependent on personal power, rather on Divine flow.

## The 4th Chakra

The egoic structures of the first three Chakras are separated from the higher Chakras by an energetic veil known as the Knot of Vishnu. Until the ego is able to let go and allow the higher Self to run the life, a barrier exists that keeps the first three Chakras separate. As the individual consciousness evolves and holds a higher vibration, the knot loosens and the higher consciousness and the higher Self take command. The 4th Chakra plays a major role in this evolution. It is the reason so many mystical paths emphasize devotional aspects such as "loving compassion," "devotion to the Master," "the love of Christ," etc. The 4th Chakra holds the key to the integration of spiritual development and to the development of the 6th and 7th states of consciousness. This Chakra is all about love. Before the dawn of higher consciousness, the personal love aspect and the hurts that have resulted in relationships can block the flow. In many ways, the 4th Chakra is composed of two facets, the personal love — the personal heart — and the universal love and compassion that comprise the spiritual heart. As the Knot of Vishnu dissolves the spiritual heart begins to flow its energies throughout the system.

The 4th Chakra holds many keys for both spiritual development, but also for healing. The ability to flow the energy of the 4th Chakra to various regions is an important part of the most healing form of Yoga asana practice (see

Chapter 6). The fourth Chakra is the seat of love. In Ayurveda, as in many traditional medicines, it is known that "love heals all." Why? Because love is in its essence the wholeness of the underlying field out of which creation arises.

Love is the stirring of consciousness in the depths of the ocean that creates a vortex and pulls everything toward it. It is pure consciousness in motion with an attractive power that can pull two souls together from the ends of the earth. Being the ocean of consciousness in its essential nature — the source of life made to flow and magnetize — it carries with it the healing energy and organizing power of the entire field of consciousness. It conveys the essence of life, of life force and of wholeness wherever it is directed. In enlivens, rejuvenates, soothes and repairs any area of the life or the body. Love is experienced as that bliss that occurs when we "fall in love." The bliss of love stirring within the heart is the movement of the bliss value of consciousness as it flows through the 4$^{th}$ Chakra.

Love heals all because it draws the power of consciousness to wherever it is directed. It is health in motion. The ocean of consciousness is the source of health, and love is the current stirring in the ocean. It is essentially consciousness *in motion*. Wherever it flows it carries wholeness, and wholeness heals.

Love is symbolized by the rose. Those familiar with the causal signature of plants (their highest vibrational overtones) know that the signature of the rose is love. It is not coincidence that roses have come to be used as an expression of love in popular culture. In ancient times there were species of rose for every ailment known to man. One rose will bring out the compassion aspect of love; another will bring out the trust aspect; and so forth. The rose family was known to be able to heal any ailment because it communicates love, and love *does* heal all.

This has great import for the development of Yogic practices because the ability to flow energy through the 4$^{th}$ Chakra freely will lead to powerful healing abilities. It only requires the proper method and education. The utilization of the 4$^{th}$ Chakra becomes a powerful tool for health and for our understanding of Yoga and Ayurveda.


## Chakras 5 – 7: The Upper System

The higher Chakras generally deal with more spiritual aspects of human existence and have more relevance in higher states of consciousness. Here is their description:

5.  *The 5$^{th}$ Chakra:* This is commonly associated with speech and speaking up but essentially it is the creative will and the will to be creative through sound and speech. The will to create in the world using speech and sound is part of an esoteric knowledge of how to create effects from the subtlest levels of consciousness utilizing vibration or sound. It is the more mundane aspects of the 5$^{th}$ Chakra that give it the sense of assertiveness in speaking up for oneself that is commonly associated with this energy center.

6.  *The 6$^{th}$ Chakra:* This Chakra is commonly called the "third eye." When the 6$^{th}$ Chakra becomes fully energized and functional, it allows one to have intuitive insight and also clairvoyant sight. It allows one to see the energetic aura and to be able to maximize intuition. It gives subtle perception as well as deep perception into people and their energetic workings.

7.  *The 7$^{th}$ Chakra:* Our center of wisdom and our direct contact with the higher spiritual vibrations comes through the 7$^{th}$ Chakra. It is thought that once opened enlightenment is attained. In reality, because it operates on the level of the Pranamaya Kosha and not on the higher spiritual levels, it does not always give enlightenment upon its opening. It does bring a strong connection with the Universal.

## Ama

As storehouses of energy and information, the Chakras are subject to toxic or polluting effects from trauma, draining relationships, and energetically toxic environments. The concept of Ama is the Ayurvedic view of toxins. Note that the common definition of Ama in most Ayurvedic texts is the residual from the improper digestion of food. Maldigestion of *anything* — food, emotions, thoughts, energies — leaves an identical residual that can block the proper projection of perfect health from the templates stored in the higher planes. It can block the flow of consciousness.

Energetic Ama is analogous to the concept of cellular memory. Those memories, and the energies they hold, stand in the way of the individual flowing Prana, energy and consciousness through the Chakras. This energy loss impairs the flow of energy into the physical organs and can eventually result in damage, disease and disability. The key point of Yogic practices and their relation to health and Ayurveda, comes from this understanding of the Chakras.

Yogi practices clear emotional, mental and energetic Ama from the Chakras and allow the Prana (energy/consciousness) to be able to flow. This enlivens the physical health and allows for deeper states of meditation and ultimately aids the growth and evolution of the individual. Yogic practices operate mainly on the Pranamaya Kosha and do so by clearing the energetic Ama and the tightly held emotions and mental patterns that get "lodged" there. This freeing allows the individual to develop and grow without the hindrances.

In essence, the correct understanding is that Yogic practices are *preparation for meditation*. They are not required for reaching Samadhi. They aid us integrating Samadhi into our daily experience. They help make permanent the experience of the fourth state of consciousness, thus promoting the development of the fifth state of consciousness. In other words, Yogic practices speed the integration of higher consciousness. But they are not necessary. They are not the means to higher consciousness.

As we have pointed out, an intimate relationship exists between the continued growth and evolution of the individual and health. Experience of Samadhi (the fourth state of consciousness) will allow for a loosening of the energetic Ama and will eventually clear it. But Yogic practices can also benefit in accelerating the clearing. When that occurs, a more clear and direct contact with the underlying field of energy and intelligence is established, and we are healthier and livelier.

The health aspect of Yoga and its relationship with Ayurveda comes from our understanding of the Chakra system. From that relationship develops a means or practice or series of techniques that purify the Chakras of Ama. As each Chakra has its connection with the Dosha and Subdoshas, we then have powerful tools for utilizing Yoga as an Ayurvedic treatment modality. With this understanding, we will be able to complete the theoretical underpinnings of the whole system of healing in the next chapter. Then we can introduce the Ayurvedic Yoga techniques that result in the purification and development toward health and enlightenment.

To complete our understanding of the Chakras, we present on the following pages the details of the Chakras. (Many thanks to Anodea Judith in her writings on the Chakras for some of the relationships with psychological issues.)

# The First Chakra

| | |
|---|---|
| **Name:** Muladhara (root) | **Mahabhuta:** Space |
| **Dosha:** Vata | **Subdosha:** Apana Vata |
| **Purpose:** Foundation | **Color:** Red |
| **Location:** Base of Spine / Coccygeal Plexus | **Nature:** Ego-based / Survival - based / Security-based |
| **Orientation:** Self-preservation | **Planet:** Saturn |
| **Psychological Issues:**<br>• Roots<br>• Grounding<br>• Trust<br>• Appropriate boundaries<br>• Family Stability<br>• Prosperity (in the sense of possessing structures)<br>• Security<br>• Belonging | **Balanced Characteristics:**<br>• Good health<br>• Vitality<br>• Well-grounded<br>• Comfortable in body<br>• Trust in the world<br>• Ability to relax and be still<br>• Right Livelihood<br>• Feeling of safety and security |
| **Illusion:** "I don't have the right to be here and to have the things I want..." | **Imbalanced Characteristics:**<br>Fear and anxiety |
| **Deficiency:**<br>• Disconnection from body<br>• Notably underweight<br>• Fearful, anxious, restless<br>• Poor focus and discipline<br>• Poor boundaries<br>• Chronic disorganization | **Excess:**<br>• Obesity, overeating<br>• Hoarding, material fixation<br>• Greed<br>• Sluggish, lazy, tired<br>• Addiction to security<br>• Fear of change<br>• Rigid boundaries |
| **Physical Manifestations**<br>• Colon disorders<br>• Disorders of the anus<br>• Disorders of bone and teeth<br>• Disorders of the legs, feet, knees, buttocks<br>• Eating disorders<br>• Frequent illness<br>• Osteoarthritis | **Healing Strategies:**<br>• Ayurvedic Yoga<br>• Effortless meditation<br>• Reconnect with body (Abhyanga, Panchakarma, dance, weight-lifting, etc.)<br>• Utilize sense of touch (Abhyanga, Panchakarma, massage)<br>• Overcome illusions with affirmations and meditation |

# The Second Chakra

| | |
|---|---|
| **Name:** Swadhisthana (sweetness) | **Mahabhuta:** Water |
| **Dosha:** Kapha and Vata | **Subdosha:** Avalambhaka Kapha & Apana Vata |
| **Purpose:** Connection / Emotional Flow / Enjoyment (pleasure) | **Color:** Orange |
| **Location:** Lower Abdomen / Sacral Plexus / Lumbar Spine | **Nature:** Ego-based / Survival-based / Emotional Connection / Bliss (pleasure) |
| **Orientation:** Self-gratification | **Planet:** Moon (connection / emotion) & Venus (pleasure / desire / enjoyment / abundance) |
| **Psychological Issues:**<br>• Emotions and emotional flow<br>• Sexuality<br>• Desire<br>• Passion<br>• Pleasure<br>• Need<br>• Abundance | **Balanced Characteristics:**<br>• Emotional intelligence<br>• Ability to experience pleasure<br>• Nurturance of self and others<br>• Ability to change and flow<br>• Healthy boundaries<br>• Graceful movements<br>• Abundant / Wealthy |
| **Illusion:** "I don't have the right to feel…" | **Imbalanced Characteristic:** Codependency, Addiction, Rigidity, Attachment, Lack of Abundance |
| **Deficiency:**<br>• Rigidity in the body and attitudes<br>• Inability to enjoy life<br>• Frigidity or fear of sex<br>• Poor social skills<br>• Denial of pleasure<br>• Excessive boundaries<br>• Fear of emotions<br>• Fear of change<br>• Lack of desire, passion, excitement | **Excess:**<br>• Ruled by emotions (crisis junkies, hysteria)<br>• Sexual addiction and acting out<br>• Pleasure addiction (including food)<br>• Excessively strong emotions<br>• Excessively sensitive / emotional<br>• Poor boundaries<br>• Seductive manipulation<br>• Emotional dependency<br>• Obsessive attachment |
| **Physical Manifestations**<br>• Disorders of reproductive organs<br>• Urogenital disorders<br>• Menstrual disorders<br>• Sexual dysfunction<br>• Low back, knee trouble or lack of flexibility<br>• Deadened senses – loss of appetite for food, sex, life | **Healing Strategies:**<br>• Ayurvedic Yoga<br>• Effortless Meditation<br>• Movement therapy (tai chi, dancing, belly dancing)<br>• Emotional release OR containment<br>• Abhyanga<br>• Ayurvedic spa treatments (facials, milk baths, etc.)<br>• Ayurvedic Counseling<br>• Aromatherapy |

# The Third Chakra

| | |
|---|---|
| **Name:** Manipura (lustrous gem) | **Mahabhuta:** Fire |
| **Dosha:** Pitta | **Subdosha:** Ranjaka Pitta |
| **Purpose:** Transformation | **Color:** Yellow |
| **Location:** Solar Plexus | **Nature:** Ego-based / Survival-based / Evaluative (Self Rating) / Personal power to affect one's world |
| **Orientation:** Self-definition | **Planet:** Mars (action to accomplish and defend) and Sun (ego) |
| **Psychological Issues:**<br>• Self-esteem<br>• Personal Power<br>• Autonomy<br>• Individuation<br>• Will and drive to accomplish | **Balanced Characteristics:**<br>• Responsible, reliable<br>• Balanced, effective will<br>• Good self-esteem<br>• Confidence<br>• Appropriate self-discipline<br>• In the right place at the right time |
| **Illusion:** "I don't have the right to be independent or powerful… / I am worthless OR more important than others…" | **Imbalanced Characteristic:** Low self-esteem / Guilt / Shame / Arrogance |
| **Deficiency:**<br>• Weak will<br>• Easily manipulated<br>• Poor self-discipline and follow-through<br>• Low self-esteem<br>• Collapsed middle<br>• Attraction to stimulants<br>• Passive<br>• Unreliable | **Excess:**<br>• Aggressive<br>• Need to be right<br>• Dominating, controlling<br>• Manipulative, power hungry<br>• Attraction to sedatives<br>• Stubbornness<br>• Driving ambition (Type A)<br>• Competitive<br>• Arrogant<br>• Hyperactive |
| **Physical Manifestations**<br>• Poor digestion<br>• Eating disorders<br>• Ulcers<br>• Hypoglycemia<br>• Diabetes<br>• Hypertension (Pitta type)<br>• Disorders of stomach, pancreas, gall bladder, liver<br>• Chronic fatigue<br>• Skin disorders<br>• Allergic disorders | **Healing Strategies:**<br>• Ayurvedic Yoga<br>• Effortless meditation<br>• Deep relaxation (Shirodhara, meditation)<br>• Vigorous exercise (aerobics, martial arts, sit-ups (deficiency))<br>• Ayurvedic Counseling re: self-worth, shame and ego strength<br>• Virechana (laxative therapy) to decrease Pitta (in excess) |

# The Fourth Chakra

| | |
|---|---|
| **Name:** Anahata (unstruck) | **Mahabhuta:** Fire |
| **Dosha:** Pitta | **Subdosha:** Sadhaka Pitta |
| **Purpose:** Love | **Color:** Green |
| **Location:** Personal Heart - Center of Chest (between the nipples) Sacred or Divine Heart (Higher Self-Connect) – 4 finger-widths above | **Nature:** Both ego-based and spirit-based /Love-nature |
| **Orientation:** Acceptance (of self and others) | **Planet:** Venus (Personal Heart) and Jupiter (Sacred Heart) |
| **Psychological Issues:**<ul><li>Love</li><li>Compassion</li><li>Self-love</li><li>Vulnerability</li><li>Intimacy</li><li>Devotion</li><li>Contentment</li><li>Fulfillment</li></ul> | **Balanced Characteristics:**<ul><li>Compassionate</li><li>Loving</li><li>Empathetic</li><li>Self-loving</li><li>Altruistic</li><li>Contented</li><li>Fulfilled</li><li>Blissful</li></ul> |
| **Illusion:** "I don't have the right to love and be loved…" | **Imbalanced Characteristic:** Walled-off, uncompassionate, unloving, coldness, grief |
| **Deficiency:**<ul><li>Antisocial, withdrawn, cold</li><li>Critical, judgmental of self or others</li><li>Loneliness</li><li>Fear of intimacy</li><li>Lack of empathy</li><li>Narcissism</li><li>Resentful</li><li>Walled-off</li></ul> | **Excess (Personal Heart Center):**<ul><li>Inability to discriminate</li><li>Demanding</li><li>Martyrdom</li><li>Hurt</li></ul> |
| **Physical Manifestations**<ul><li>Disorders of the heart, thymus</li><li>Lungs Disorders</li><li>Disorders of the breast</li><li>Upper arms</li><li>Sunken chest</li><li>Circulation problems</li><li>Asthma</li></ul> | **Healing Strategies:**<ul><li>Ayurvedic Yoga</li><li>Effortless meditation</li><li>Utilize sense of touch (Abhyanga, Panchakarma, massage)</li><li>Ayurvedic Counseling</li><li>Behavioral Rasayanas (connecting with children or pets)</li><li>Aromatherapy</li></ul> |

# The Fifth Chakra

| | |
|---|---|
| **Name:** Vissudha (Purification) | **Mahabhuta:** Air |
| **Dosha:** Vata | **Subdosha:** Udana Vata |
| **Purpose:** Communication / Intellectual Creativity | **Color:** Bright Blue |
| **Location:** Throat | **Nature:** Spirit-based / Creative / The Will to Create Through Speech |
| **Orientation:** Self-expression | **Planet:** Mercury |
| **Psychological Issues:**<ul><li>Communication</li><li>Creativity</li><li>Listening</li><li>Resonance</li><li>Finding one's own voice</li><li>Creating effects through speech</li></ul> | **Balanced Characteristics:**<ul><li>Clear communication</li><li>Diplomatic</li><li>Lives creatively</li><li>Resonant voice</li><li>Good listener</li></ul> |
| **Illusion:** "I don't have the right to speak, to express…" | **Imbalanced Characteristic:** Unable to speak up or speak for oneself / Lies |
| **Deficiency:**<ul><li>Fear of speaking</li><li>Small, weak voice</li><li>Difficulty with putting feelings into words</li><li>Introversion</li><li>Tone deaf</li><li>Poor rhythm</li></ul> | **Excess:**<ul><li>Excessive talking</li><li>Using talking as a defense</li><li>Inability to listen</li><li>Poor auditory comprehension</li><li>Gossiping</li><li>Dominating conversations</li></ul> |
| **Physical Manifestations**<ul><li>Sore throat</li><li>Ear problems</li><li>Hoarseness</li><li>Voice disorders</li><li>Lymphatic congestion or toxicity</li><li>Tightness of jaw</li><li>TMJ</li><li>Allergies</li></ul> | **Healing Strategies:**<ul><li>Ayurvedic Yoga</li><li>Effortless meditation</li><li>Utilize sense of sound (chanting, singing, toning)</li><li>Silence (for excessive)</li><li>Teach listening and communication skills</li><li>Voice lessons</li><li>Journaling</li><li>Nasya</li><li>Ayurvedic Counseling</li></ul> |

# The Sixth Chakra

| | |
|---|---|
| **Name:** Ajna (to perceive and command) | **Mahabhuta:** Fire |
| **Dosha:** Pitta | **Subdosha:** Alochaka Pitta |
| **Purpose:** To See Into Things | **Color:** Indigo |
| **Location:** Forehead (Third Eye) | **Nature:** Spirit-based /Perception of Archetypal (Causal) Patterning / Clairvoyance |
| **Orientation:** Self-reflection | **Planet:** Jupiter |
| **Psychological Issues:**<br>• Insight<br>• Intuition<br>• Imagination<br>• Visualization<br>• Dreams<br>• Vision<br>• Memory | **Balanced Characteristics:**<br>• Perceptive<br>• Intuitive<br>• Good memory<br>• Able to access and remember dreams<br>• Able to think symbolically<br>• Able to visualize |
| **Illusion:** "I don't have the right to see…" | **Imbalanced Characteristic:**<br>Illusion / Lack of Insight |
| **Deficiency:**<br>• Poor vision<br>• Poor memory<br>• Difficulty imaging alternatives<br>• Difficulty visualizing<br>• Denial (can't see what is going on)<br>• Rigidity (one true and only true way) | **Excess:**<br>• Delusions<br>• Obsessions<br>• Nightmares<br>• Hallucinations<br>• Difficulty concentrating |
| **Physical Manifestations**<br>• Vision problems<br>• Headaches<br>• Head pressure | **Healing Strategies:**<br>• Effortless meditation<br>• Mandalas<br>• Color therapy<br>• Creative visualization<br>• Shirodhara<br>• Ayurvedic Counseling |

# The Seventh Chakra

| | |
|---|---|
| **Name:** Sahasrara (Thousand-fold) | **Mahabhuta:** Space |
| **Dosha:** Vata | **Subdosha:** Prana Vata |
| **Purpose:** Liberation | **Color:** Violet |
| **Location:** Crown of Head | **Nature:** Spirit-based, Higher Consciousness / Universal / Spiritual |
| **Orientation:** Self-knowledge | **Planet:** Ketu |
| **Psychological Issues:**<br>• Transcendence<br>• Higher Power<br>• Union<br>• Letting go of belief systems<br>• Integration | **Balanced Characteristics:**<br>• Ability to integrate experience<br>• Wise<br>• Open-minded<br>• Spiritually connected |
| **Illusion:** "I don't have the right to spirituality, to be free from attachment…" | **Imbalanced Characteristic:** Attachment / Materialistic |
| **Deficiency:**<br>• Spiritual cynicism<br>• Difficulty learning from experience and integrating experience<br>• Rigid belief systems<br>• Apathy<br>• Excessive focus on lower Chakra issues – materialism, greed, power over others, etc. | **Excess:**<br>• Dissociation from the body<br>• Confusion<br>• Spaciness<br>• Spiritual addiction |
| **Physical Manifestations**<br>• Headaches<br>• Brain tumors | **Healing Strategies:**<br>• Effortless meditation<br>• Ayurvedic Yoga to ground spirit into the physical<br>• Psychotherapy focused on beliefs and transpersonal psychology<br>• Shirodhara |

# Yoga and Ayurveda

*Chapter 5*

DOSHA, CHAKRA & PLANET

# Dosha, Chakra and Planet

The premise of this book has been that health is dependent on our contact with Wholeness. The experience of Union (Yoga) known as Samadhi or transcendental consciousness forms the basis for the enlivenment of health, growth and evolution. This development can be hampered if there is no strong contact with the underlying field of consciousness (i.e., the light is dim) or if there is energetic or physical Ama (i.e., dust and debris on the film). In order to project perfect health onto the movie screen of life, we must also attend to the film that forms the template for the movie. If the film is warped or distorted, the physical form will also be malformed.

Balance in the "templates" is created by the *Doshas* in Ayurvedic terminology. Many an Ayurvedic aficionado has been surprised to learn the meaning of this term, as they see the body being "made up" of the Doshas. Dosha means "impurity." The Doshas represent the combinations formed from the fundamental elements that arise out of the underlying field. They are in a virtual form that guides the unfolding and functioning of the human physiology. Yet, because they do not contain the fullness and purity of the entire unified field, they are "impure" and therefore called Doshas. They are composed of fundamental elements. These fundamental elements or *Mahabhutas* are:

1. Space
2. Air
3. Fire
4. Water
5. Earth

Space is not as some translations suggest "ether." What the ancients cognized as the fundamentals of creation was beyond subtle energies. They cognized the unfolding of creation from the inception of space and time — beyond all energy and form. What the ancient sages were referencing is one and the same as that which modern quantum physicists describe. They portray creation arising from virtual particles that form the template for physical creation. "Virtual particles" are subatomic particles that have no physical existence — they are potential or "virtual" in their nature. They are the potentials that are created in the unified field, as the nonmaterial or energetic aspects of the field begin to stir. Physicists describe five possible spin types to the virtual particles. These correspond perfectly with the Mahabhutas. The first of these, the Graviton, is responsible for the warp in space-time that we call gravity. It is an expression of space, not ether.

The Mahabhutas are the first virtual patterning that comes out of the underlying field. They combine to form the Doshas as follows:

1. *Vata* — Space and Air
2. *Pitta* — Fire and Water
3. *Kapha* — Water and Earth

Again, each of these is a patterning of the potentials of the underlying field that are missing the "Whole." This absence of all the qualities of the unified field is what makes the "impure" nature of the Doshas. While the Doshas are often conceived of as energies, they actually are at the level of creation that precedes energy. They guide the unfolding of energies, flows, movements and transformations in the body. They are not those energies and flows.

While popular culture emphasizes the nature of the Doshas in guiding the development of one's constitution or "body type," they guide all of the body's functioning and, more important, its state of balance. Body types can be organized along the guiding principles of the Doshas:

1. Vata — thin, small, short, tiny, light, airy nature
2. Pitta — muscular, angular, medium, intense, fiery nature
3. Kapha — large, tall, stout, heavy, earthy nature

Body type, though, only tells us what imbalances we will be more prone to, on average. When the body is in balance, body type tells us what types of food and routines can best keep it in proper balance. For example, a Vata type that is full of lightness and airiness needs foods that are heavy and grounding. Otherwise they are prone to accumulating more of the "air" or "space" quality. In that accumulation, they end up with symptoms such as "spaciness" or emaciation or dry skin (air creates wind that dries out the body as it blows on it constantly). A list of typical characteristics of the Doshas and some details of the body types are listed on the next pages.

# Vata Dosha

- Composed of the elements (*Mahabhutas*): space and air
- Qualities:
    - light
    - dry
    - coarse
    - rough
    - dark
    - changeable
    - moveable
    - subtle
    - cold
    - clear
- Body Type: light build, thin
- Handshake: cold, thin, weak (the wet fish)
- Psychology in Balance: enthusiastic, vivacious, talkative
- Psychology Out of Balance: anxious, fearful, nervous, unstable
- Foods that Aggravate: cold, raw, rough (salads), dry foods (beans), light foods (popcorn)
- Foods that Pacify: warm, unctuous (oily), heavy
- Colors: dark blue, black, dark brown
- Season: fall, early winter
- Time of Day: 2-6 AM or PM
- Location in Physiology: colon, joints, inside of bones, nervous system
- Major Functions in Physiology: movement, transportation, communication

# Pitta Dosha

- Composed of the Mahabhutas: fire and water
- Qualities:
  - hot
  - sharp
  - pungent
  - intense
  - flowing (but grounded)
  - sour
  - oily (slightly)
- Body Type: medium build, muscular
- Handshake: crushing grip, warm hand
- Psychology in Balance: focused, generous, goal-oriented, analytical
- Psychology Out of Balance: too intense, aggressive, egotistical
- Foods that Aggravate: hot, spicy (chilies, ginger), burning or acidic (vinegar, citrus)
- Foods that Pacify: cool, soothing foods with sweet, bitter and astringent tastes
- Colors: orange, light intense blue
- Season: summer
- Time of Day: 10-2 AM or PM
- Location in Physiology: liver, small intestine, skin
- Major Functions in Physiology: digestion, metabolism and transformation

# Kapha Dosha

- Composed of the Mahabhutas: earth and water
- Qualities:
    - unctuous (oily)
    - slimy
    - cool
    - moist
    - sticky
    - heavy
    - stable
    - strong
    - soft
- Body type: large build
- Handshake: soft puffy pillow
- Psychology in Balance: jovial, sweet, loving, easy-going
- Psychology Out of Balance: dull, lethargic, resistant
- Foods that Aggravate: sweet, heavy (cheesecake), oily, substantial (meat=oily, heavy)
- Foods that Pacify: Light, dry foods with pungent, bitter and astringent tastes
- Colors: white, light brown
- Season: winter, early spring
- Time of Day: 6-10 AM or PM
- Location in Physiology: chest, low back
- Function in Physiology: structure, strength (immunity), lubrication

It can be useful to study the body types, but the importance of that is way overblown in modern culture. So few of us are in balance that its practical relevance is hard to find. Any body type can have any Doshic imbalance. Most of us have more than one type of imbalance at the same time. To base all diet and lifestyle recommendations on body type is missing the boat for the vast majority of people. Here are some examples of the types of imbalances associated with the Doshas:

## Signs of Vata Dosha Imbalance

| | |
|---|---|
| Appetite | Variable, with little consistency from one day to the next |
| Digestion | Poor, with variable digestive capacity |
| Stool | Hard, dry, dark, prone to constipation |
| Urine | Light in color, frequent urination |
| Menstruation | Irregular cycles with severe cramping and scanty blood flow |
| Movement | Cramping or spastic movements |
| Physical Activity | Addicted to movement |
| Sleep | Light or prone to insomnia |
| Voice | Weak, tires easily, prone to hoarseness |
| Speech | Fast, erratic |
| Skin | Dry, flaky |
| Hair | Dry, brittle |
| Joints | Cracking |
| Relationships | Shy, dependent, stressed |
| | |
| | VATA DISEASES / CONDITIONS |
| | <ul><li>Arthritis</li><li>High or low blood pressure</li><li>Bladder/urinary disorders</li><li>Headaches (tension)</li><li>Dizziness</li><li>Tinnitus (ringing in the ears)</li><li>Gas and bloating</li><li>Chronic fatigue</li><li>Fibromyalgia</li></ul> |

# Signs of Pitta Dosha Imbalance

| | |
|---|---|
| Appetite | Too strong, becomes irritable when skipping a meal |
| Digestion | Too strong, easily aggravated by spicy foods |
| Stool | Soft, loose, burning, lighter in color; frequent bowel movements or diarrhea |
| Urine | Bright yellow, often in excess |
| Menstruation | Regular but may have heavy bleeding or longer period due to internal heat |
| Movement | Determined stride |
| Physical Activity | Overdoes vigorous exercise and becomes too competitive at sports |
| Sleep | Light, early morning awakenings |
| Voice | Loud, often piercing |
| Speech | Sharp and direct |
| Skin | Delicate, oily skin; prone to acne and rashes |
| Hair | Premature graying and hair loss common |
| Relationships | Overly intense, manipulative, stubborn, jealous, egotistical, demeaning |
| | |
| | PITTA DISEASES / CONDITIONS |
| | <ul><li>Heartburn</li><li>Hot flashes</li><li>Skin rashes</li><li>Psoriasis</li><li>Ulcers</li><li>Inflammation</li><li>Canker sores</li><li>Diarrhea</li><li>Liver disorders</li><li>Bloodshot eyes</li><li>Excessive hunger and thirst</li></ul> |

# Signs of Kapha Dosha Imbalance

| | |
|---|---|
| Appetite | Not strong; often not hungry upon awakening |
| Digestion | Digestive fire often weak; slow metabolism |
| Stool | Well-formed, often with an oily coat |
| Urine | White and foamy; infrequent elimination |
| Menstruation | Regular but prone to water retention and clotting |
| Movement | Sluggish |
| Physical Activity | Capable of vigorous activity but tends to avoid physical exertion |
| Sleep | Deep sleep, often snores, oversleeps |
| Voice | Thick, melodious, low |
| Speech | Slow and deliberate |
| Skin | Oily, smooth, cool |
| Hair | Thick, oily |
| Relationships | Attached, greedy |
| | |
| | KAPHA DISEASES / CONDITIONS |
| | • Obesity<br>• Diabetes<br>• Yeast conditions<br>• Lymphatic system disorders<br>• Water retention/bloating<br>• Low thyroid function<br>• Congestive heart failure |

As can be readily seen, *any body type can have any of these imbalances*. So focusing on body type is really misleading. So few of us are in balance that the relevance of body type is hard to find. Any body type can have any Doshic imbalance, and most of us have more than one type of imbalance at the same time. To guide all diet and lifestyle recommendations from body type is a disservice for the vast majority of people.

The greatest potential for healing lies in balancing the Doshas, regardless of body type. To do that, we can use the knowledge of the Doshas to describe what is found in the natural world. When we learn one simple rule — *like increases like* — then all of nature becomes at our disposal for rebalancing the body and creating health.

"Like increases like" means that if we take a light and airy food like popcorn and put a person on a diet made up of purely popcorn, they will become even more light and airy. In other words a Vata food increases Vata in the human physiology. If we take a heavy dense food like steak and put a person on a steak diet, they become heavy and dense (they gain weight, cholesterol goes up, etc.). The Kapha food increases Kapha in the physiology.

It is not just food, though, that has Doshic properties. Once this is realized we are able to tap into one of the most important aspects of the Doshas — that the knowledge of the Doshas puts all of nature at our disposal and turns it into our personal pharmacy.

## The Universal Pharmacy

The natural laws that govern the Doshas provide us the ability to rethink our concept of medicine. If you can describe any substance in the universe in terms of the Doshas, it can become your medicine — you know its impact on the human physiology. The Doshas guide the unfolding of the human body, and the quality of a substance will affect the physiology according to it Doshic properties. Take a color like dark blue.

It is close to the color of space and thus has that cool Vata quality — Vata being made of space and air qualities. Thus, if we are experiencing too many fiery Pitta emotions, wearing dark blue can help the mind-body to "chill." We have in this example reinvented color therapy. The ancient Ayurvedic physicians knew this and utilized it as a matter of course, without having to give it the name "color therapy."

It is not just colors that are part of the universal pharmacy. Any substance in creation that we describe becomes a part of our armamentarium. Take a song for example. It can be sweet and melodious (Kapha in nature), harsh and aggressive (think punk rock — Pitta in nature) or fast-paced, quick, lively and stimulating (think the Charleston — Vata in nature). Each type of music will increase that Dosha in the body.

In this manner, Ayurveda contains all of the natural therapies from color therapy to music therapy to aromatherapy to gem therapy to a detailed understanding of diet and herbs. On a superficial level, this knowledge is applied to the practice of Yoga to temper the style to be either "restorative" (grounding and relaxing — Vata pacifying), "Vinyasa flow" (stimulating and more strenuous — Kapha pacifying) or a style described as "cooling" (think Moon salutation — Pitta pacifying). While there is some value to this approach, it completely misses the mark of the healing potential of Yoga as described by Patanjali and Charaka. Those who utilize Yoga to heal understand that the value is not in the style of the practice, rather in the inner work that is done in the posture. This inner work relates to the subtle energies and the subtle flows that ultimately profoundly influence the Doshas and their balance.

In order to understand how the subtle flows and the Chakras relate to the Doshas, we must have a detailed understanding of the *functions* that the Doshas rule and their relationship to the Subdoshas.

**THE FUNCTIONS OF THE DOSHAS**

The ancient sages were not so naïve as to think that the body was composed of "air," "fire" and "earth." They saw that the body's functions *patterned* after these. The Doshas guide function and creation. They are part of the organizing power of the unified field of consciousness. It is in the proper functioning that we find the proper balance, and it is in imbalance that functioning becomes improper. Charaka and others outlined the functioning of each of the Doshas. These are detailed in the following table:

# Dosha Functions
# According to the Ancients

| BALANCED VATA FUNCTIONS | BALANCED PITTA FUNCTIONS | BALANCED KAPHA FUNCTIONS |
|---|---|---|
| Enthusiasm | Sight | Unctuousness |
| Expiration | Digestion | Binding |
| Inhalation | Heat | Firmness |
| Movement | Thirst | Strength |
| Balanced Development of Dhatus (tissues) | Hunger | Potency |
| Balanced Malas (waste products) | Softness | Heaviness |
| | Luster | Forbearance |
| | Cheerfulness | Patience |
| | Good Intellect | Absence of Greed |

A more modern and simple view would be to take each Dosha and assign it three categories of functions. In this way, we can delve deeper into the physiology and how it works. Here are the major functions from a modern perspective:

1. *Vata — Movement, Communication, Transportation:* This means movement of limbs, breathing and musculature, which differs from transportation. Transportation refers to the movement of substances within the body, ranging from the transporting of food along the digestive tract to the transporting of biochemicals in and out cells. Communication is the movement and flow of energy and nerve impulses. Vata rules the nervous system and is responsible for all intercellular communication. All nervous system functions are affected by Vata, implying that stress, worry and hurry are all related to the state of Vata in an individual.

2. *Pitta — Digestion, Metabolism, Transformation:* Digestion means the absorption, assimilation and transforming of food into energy and tissues. It is different from elimination, which is the removal of wastes (and is under the influence of Vata). Metabolism is the maintenance of body temperature on the gross level and the production of energy on the cellular level. All of the enzymatic processes in the body are under the transformation aspect of Pitta. To be able to transform all the aspects of food into living tissue is the role of Pitta.

3. *Kapha — Structure, Strength, Lubrication:* Pitta supplies the building blocks to Kapha. Kapha forms the cohesion and binding together of the building blocks and is responsible for the human frame. It is the structure or substance of the body. It is responsible for strength. Strength in the eyes of the sages was not just muscular strength, rather the strength to resist disease (immunity). The lubrication aspect of Kapha is in the joints, the lining of the stomach, the

moistening of the lungs and the protection of the brain (cerebrospinal fluid).

The body is in essence a series of functions and processes. The Doshas guide those processes. In order to affect those processes and their domains of functioning, we must go beyond a superficial approach to Yoga practice. We must have a more direct connection to the inner workings of the body. In order to understand how this can be done, we must add one more level of understanding — the Subdoshas.

The Subdoshas are specific areas of functioning of the Doshas. They have an intimate connection with the Chakra system and that relationship holds the key to utilizing Yoga to heal. Each Subdosha has a location and specific area of function and typical types of diseases and conditions that result when they are out of balance. The following tables elucidate these:

# Vata Subdoshas

| SUBDOSHA | LOCATION | FUNCTIONS | COMMON CONDITIONS |
|---|---|---|---|
| Prana Vata | Brain<br>Head<br>Throat<br>Heart<br>Respiratory organs | "The breath that nourishes the brain"<br>Clarity of mind and reasoning<br>Memory<br>Enthusiasm<br>Sneezing<br>Belching<br>Respiration | Anxiety<br>Worry<br>Overactive mind<br>Insomnia<br>Hiccups<br>Asthma<br>Blocked nasal passages<br>Lung diseases |
| Udana Vata | Throat<br>Lungs | Speech<br>Singing<br>Motivation<br>Effort<br>Swallowing<br>Breathing | Sore Throat<br>Allergies<br>Sinus congestion<br>Difficulty speaking up for oneself<br>Fatigue<br>Speech disorders |
| Samana Vata | Stomach<br>Intestines | "The breath that fans the fire of digestion"<br>Peristalsis | Reflux disease<br>Weak digestion<br>Migraine headaches<br>Anorexia<br>Bloating |
| Apana Vata | Colon<br>Bladder<br>Navel<br>Thighs<br>Groin<br>Reproductive system<br>Rectum | Downward flow of energy<br>Elimination of wastes<br>Sexual discharge<br>Menstruation | Constipation<br>Irritable Bowel Syndrome<br>Colitis<br>Diarrhea<br>Flatulence<br>Low back pain<br>Hip pain<br>Knee pain<br>Hemorrhoids<br>Menstrual problems<br>Sexual dysfunction |
| Vyana Vata | Diffused throughout the body<br>The microcirculation<br>The peripheral nervous system | Circulation<br>Blood pressure<br>Sense of touch | Hypertension<br>Hypotension<br>Tension headaches<br>Heart arrhythmias<br>Nervous system diseases |

# Pitta Subdoshas

| SUBDOSHA | LOCATION | FUNCTIONS | COMMON CONDITIONS |
|---|---|---|---|
| Pachaka Pitta | Stomach<br>Small intestine | "Cooks" the food<br><br>Transforms food<br><br>Separates waste from food | Ulcers<br>Digestive weakness<br>Heartburn<br>Hyperacidity<br>Stomachache |
| Ranjaka Pitta | Liver<br>Gallbladder | "Colors the blood" (responsible for the formation of the blood)<br><br>Manufacture of Proteins<br>Regulation of blood sugar<br>Cholesterol | Skin rashes<br>Allergies,<br>Hyperlipidemia<br>Anemia<br>Jaundice<br>Irritability<br>Early Morning Awakening<br>Hot flashes<br>PMS |
| Sadhaka Pitta | Heart | "The fire of the heart"<br>Passion<br>Fulfillment<br>Contentment<br>Memory<br>Intelligence | Discontent<br>"Your heart not being in what you are doing"<br>Difficulty making decisions<br>Loss of passion<br>Sadness<br>Depression<br>Memory loss,<br>Psychiatric disturbance,<br>Heart disease |
| Alochaka Pitta | Eyes | Sight<br>Insight<br>Ability to see into things<br><br>The third eye | Eye irritation<br>Eye strain<br>Bloodshot eyes<br>Vision problems<br>Lack of insight<br>Strain on the third eye |
| Bhrajaka Pitta | Diffused throughout the body<br><br>The skin | The metabolism and transformations that takes place in the skin<br><br>The glow of the skin | Skin disease<br>Boils<br>Acne<br>Rashes |

# Kapha Subdoshas

| SUBDOSHA | LOCATION | FUNCTIONS | COMMON CONDITIONS |
|---|---|---|---|
| Kledaka Kapha | Stomach | Lubricates the stomach<br><br>Moistening and initial digestion of food. | Dull digestion<br>Ulcers |
| Avalambaka Kapha | Lumbar region<br>Chest<br>Heart<br>Lungs | Supports lumbar region and also the heart<br><br>Gives strength and stamina in these regions, but also in the upper torso | Back pain<br>Sciatica<br>Heart problems (physical heart)<br>Congestive heart failure<br>Asthma<br>Lethargy |
| Bodhaka Kapha | Tongue<br>Throat | Moistening the tongue<br><br>Secretion of mucous<br><br>Taste | Gum disease<br>Canker sores<br>Loss of taste<br>Lack of secretions |
| Tarpaka Kapha | Cerebrospinal fluid<br>Head | Nourishment of the mind<br><br>Integration of experience and information in the brain<br><br>Maintenance of spinal fluid | Problems integrating new information and learning from experience<br><br>Disruption in the sense of smell<br><br>Disruption of cerebrospinal fluid |
| Shleshaka Kapha | Joints | Lubrication of joints throughout the body | Joint problems<br>Joint stiffness<br>Arthritis |

The beauty of Ayurveda is that it has reliable methods of detecting imbalances in the Subdoshas long before the manifestation of disease. The use of refined observation of the pulse can give an Ayurvedic physician a clear picture of the state of the Subdoshas. The tables list "Common Conditions." These reflect more the commonly found associations with the pulse findings, rather than a comprehensive list of all conditions and diseases that can result when a Subdosha is out of balance.

## THE SUBDOSHAS AND THE CHAKRAS

In clinical experience certain Subdoshas have a major impact on the functionings of the Doshas — they tend to "rule" that Dosha. They are found to be out of balance much more frequently. In Vata Dosha the Subdosha that appears to rule its functions are Apana Vata (located in the lower abdomen). In Pitta Dosha the major Subdosha is Ranjanka (liver/gallbladder). In Kapha Dosha the ruling Subdosha is Avalambhaka Kapha (lumbar spine, chest). Clinical experience correlates with what the ancient sages labeled the "seat" of each Dosha (Vata in the colon, Pitta in the liver/small intestine, Kapha in the chest). The importance of the seat is that when that area goes out of balance it tends to throw the entire Dosha out of balance and set up the conditions for disease and dysfunction.

It is no coincidence that the major Subdoshas are at the exact placement of the major Chakras:

- Apana Vata — 1st Chakra
- Avalambhaka Kapha — 2nd Chakra
- Ranjaka Pitta — 3rd Chakra
- Sadhaka Pitta — 4th Chakra

In other words, *the major control of the Doshas comes from the Chakras.* This is the key understanding that has been missing from the knowledge of Yoga and Ayurveda. Here finally we have the key to balancing the Doshas through Yogic practices. It comes through working with the Chakras and the flow of energy through each. This gives us a powerful method for affecting balance and health through the practice of Yoga that emphasizes working energetically with the Chakras.

The Chakras are actually complex in that they have a front and back and sides and slightly different functions and associations with these. For that reason our simplified association of the four major Subdoshas with the four major Chakras is in need of some refinement. Here is a more complete understanding:

# The Chakras and the Subdoshas

| Chakra | Planet | Dosha | Disease Examples | Emotional Complex |
|---|---|---|---|---|
| 1 | Saturn | Apana Vata | *Minor:* Constipation *Major:* Arthritis | *Core:* Fear *Related:* Holding on Controlling |
| 2 | Moon / Venus | Apana Vata Avalambhaka Kapha | *Minor:* Low backache *Major:* Pelvic infections, Prostatitis, Impotence, Frigidity | *Core:* Attachment *Related:* Attachment to things rather than people |
| 3 | Mars / Sun | Ranjaka Pitta | *Minor:* Skin rash, allergies *Major:* Ulcerative Colitis, Cirrhosis | *Core:* Low Self-esteem *Related:* Competitive-ness, Egoism, Irritability, Anger |
| 4 | Venus / Jupiter | Sadhaka Pitta | *Minor:* Discontent, depression *Major:* Heart disease | *Core:* Hurt *Related:* Self-protective, unemotional |
| 5 | Mercury | Udana Vata | *Minor:* Sore Throat, Difficulty speaking up *Major:* Thyroid disease | *Core:* Unassertive-ness |
| 6 | Jupiter | Alochaka Pitta | *Minor:* Insomnia *Major:* Psychosis | *Core:* Over-intellectualizing |
| 7 | Ketu | Prana Vata | *Minor:* Headaches *Major:* Ignorance, Dementia, Inability to evolve | *Core:* Denial, particularly of spiritual development |

To understand this, we must remember that the Chakras have different aspects. Take the 2$^{nd}$ Chakra as an example. It can relate to the more emotional aspects (Apana / Moon) or to the more sensual, beauty and luxury (wealth) aspect (Avalambhaka / Venus). Note also that now we can see a connection between Vedic Astrology (Jyotish), the Chakras, and ultimately health. This is why the ancient physicians were also skilled in Vedic Astrology. Finally, we can understand how all aspects of Ayurveda, Yoga and Jyotish are connected. We can also see the necessity of integrating them into our practice and utilization of Ayurveda.

With this knowledge of the connection between the Doshas and the Chakras, we are finally ready to understand how to use Yogic practices to create health.

# Yoga and Ayurveda

*Chapter 6*

# Yogic Healing

The amazing ability the mind has to separate and categorize things gives rise to the illusion that health, spirituality and physical Yoga practices are all separate things. When consciousness is bound in the waking state it allows the mind to pretend that these things are separate. The mind in normal consciousness can create this sort of illusion. Imagine if we could only view the world through a narrow slit in a fence and only view it at one-second intervals. A cat walking by on the other side of the fence would appear as first a head, then a tail. We'd miss what was in between. We would think that a cat's head and a cat's tail were two separate things. This is the way the mind works in normal waking consciousness until our awareness is developed and the path to higher consciousness is begun.

The source of health and the source of spiritual development are one and the same. Unfortunately, most people have been deprived of a means of developing and expanding their consciousness and thus the illusions of a cat's head of health and a cat's tail of spiritual evolution are seen as very separate things. Without the development of consciousness our ability to perceive reality is hampered. We can create the illusion that these things are all separate. Without the ability to perceive reality fully, we can create all sorts of beliefs about what spirit is and what is responsible for health. This is the difference between religion and spirituality. Religion is based on belief, and spirituality is based on experience of reality. This is why the enlightened seers were referred to as "the knowers of reality." They had developed their consciousness to experience reality and to know firsthand how creation works.

This ability to perceive reality is not just being a little more awake and aware. It involves an entire shift in the wiring of the brain, and in perception and insight. Without direct experience, analogies are the only way to get a feel for this tremendous difference. The analogy presented below is drawn from developmental psychology, where the relationship between brain development and perception is clearly understood.

The father of modern developmental psychology is Jean Piaget. His work on the development of cognitive structures has influenced almost every area of psychology, from learning and cognition to child development and testing. The essence of his genius lies in a simple, yet profound recognition: It is not that a child is simply inexperienced and unlearned — a child's brain is organized differently, and children think and perceive reality differently from adults. The easiest way to describe this difference in cognitive structures is to use one of his classic experiments:

> Take a bowl that is fat, has a large diameter, but is not very tall. Take a cylinder that is thin, has a small diameter, and is tall. Then take a 6 oz. glass full of water and pour its contents in the fat bowl. Now refill the glass and pour it into the tall cylinder. Now look at both. Which has more?

How you answer that question depends on the structure and functioning of the brain and how accurately that functioning allows for a true perception of reality. Most adults will clearly state that they have the same amount of water. Now ask most 4-year-olds. Half of them will say that the bowl has more. If you ask them why, they will say it is because it is fatter. The other half will say that the cylinder has more. If you ask them why, they will say because it is taller. It does not matter how often you explain to these children that the two *appear* to be different, but are really the *same*. Experiencing pouring the same amount into each cylinder does not matter; experience and education do not matter — the child perceives them as different.

Now if you are a behaviorist and think all of life is about reinforcement, you can devise a way to reinforce the correct answer. You can bribe 4-year-olds into giving you the correct answer to the question of which has more, by giving them some cookies or some other reward. But if you pull one of them aside and ask them what they really *believe*, they will tell you one or the other really has more. They simply do not have the brain structure to be able to perceive in two dimensions. They can't take into account two variables — height and width. If you do the same experiment with 8-year-olds, you find that they give a very different answer. The vast majority of them will know that the two containers are equal. They can think in two dimensions, not because they are "smarter," rather because their brains have been wired through growth to perceive reality more fully.

Piaget made many such experiments and concluded that there are distinct stages in cognitive development. It did not matter what the I.Q. of the child was, how good his or her memory was, or how quickly they learned. Until a different style of functioning of the brain occurs, the ability to perceive more than one dimension of reality is simply not present. The 4-year-old thinks in one dimension. His or her comprehension of reality is based entirely on information from the senses, and because the perception is undeveloped, they see in one dimension. If the height dimension strikes the child as the most outstanding feature, then the cylinder has more. If the width dimension is predominant, then the bowl has more.

This is analogous to normal waking consciousness where our awareness of ourselves is overshadowed by thoughts, emotions or physical sensations. We "identify" with one or more of these to the exclusion of our awareness of ourselves as the observer of the thoughts, emotions or sensations. Until consciousness is more developed, there is this fragmentation in our perception of reality.

Suppose the world were made up of people whose brains had only developed to the 4-year-old stage. They would appear as adults, and because they could remember and learn things, no one would know the difference. But when confronted with a dilemma like the one of which container has "more," what would happen? Most likely we would see a political party develop of the "Tall-ists" and one of the "Wide-ists" and the two would never see eye-to-eye. They would have fervent arguments about why their party was right and why they should rule the country. They would believe sincerely and strongly about their views and feel uncomfortable around those who held the opposite view. They might even get into fights at times. Worse yet, they might believe so strongly in their limited perception that they would turn their beliefs into a religion and go on crusades trying to convert people to their way of believing, making others feel less worthy if they did not believe. In the most tragic case, they would wage war in the name of their beliefs, feeling it was their righteous duty.

Suppose out of the hills comes a man who has been apart from society and has developed his brain to that of an 8-year-old. The 8-year-old looks with curiosity at all the political and religious bickering and says, "No, no, no. There is no need for all of this. They are not different. They are all the same. It is the same water that goes into both. It is one and the same." The 4-year-olds would certainly be taken aback and say, "That person is crazy. Anyone can see they are different. Why would you ever believe this theoretical 'unity' garbage? It is just mystical mumbo-jumbo…"

The worlds of Ayurveda, Yoga and spirituality are very much in an analogous state. Like the cat's head and tail, the separation of these fields is part of the illusion of the mind. That illusion will persist until the brain evolves and grows and develops the ability to know and experience reality directly. Patanjali and Charaka knew this and never thought to separate health from evolution and spiritual development. In fact, if we look at the fourth verse of the very first page of the Charaka Samhita, we see this:

> When diseases appeared as impediments to spiritual pursuits, self-study, divine conduct, meditation and life itself, then the great sages having compassion for all beings gathered in the Himalayan region [to cognize Ayurveda].

Patanjali also in his first quarter references the obstacles to developing consciousness and lists several, but the first is as follows:

> The objects which disturb consciousness are *illness*, dullness, doubt, negligence, laziness, self-destructive habits, mistaken perception, ungroundedness, and instability. [Pada 1 Sutra 30]

Both Charaka and Patanjali understood that health and the development of consciousness are intimately related and that illness is a major block to contact with the source of our liveliness and energy. The purpose of Yogic practices is to clear the body of stresses and imbalances that might block the full evolution and growth of consciousness and the growth of health. In this manner illness can be prevented and evolution assured.

Yogic practices are to clear the way to "Union." They are preparation for meditation, so that we can directly contact the source of health. Illness is a major impediment that is the result of imbalances that have ripened to the point of creating physical disturbance. Utilizing Yogic practices for their maximum benefit must involve the rebalancing of the Doshas and clearing emotional, mental and energetic Ama. As we have seen, the Chakras are also the key to this entire endeavor. Rebalancing the Doshas takes place through the major Subdoshas and their control centers — the Chakras. Additionally, most of the energetic, emotional and mental Ama resides in the Chakras themselves. Yogic practices clear the Ama from the Chakras and rebalance the Doshas via the Subdoshas. In this manner, yogic practices facilitate the way to Union, wholeness and health.

The ultimate utilization of Yoga for health involves a practice that clears the Chakras of Ama, rebalances the Doshas and removes the stresses that impede meditation and spiritual development. That optimal method for this purification patterns itself after the purification therapies (Panchakarma therapies) of Ayurveda:

1. *Preparation — Softening and loosening the Ama:*
Sometimes referred to as "ripening the Ama" the
physiology must be prepared prior to the elimination.
Otherwise there is chance of actually pushing the
Ama deeper into the tissues of the body. This is like
putting some salt on an icy sidewalk — you create
some heat that starts to melt the ice and it becomes
much easier to shovel and clear. If you don't prepare
the system for the elimination of Ama it can be like
using too much force to remove a screw — you may
strip the head and make it much harder to remove.

2. *Purification — Eliminating Ama from the system:* Once
the Ama is softened and ripened it naturally moves
towards the digestive tract in the physical Kosha. It
can then be eliminated naturally, in the manner the
body eliminates wastes or foreign substances (through
purging or pushing things out the colon rapidly or
sneezing or the other natural ways the body purifies).

3. *Rebalancing — The Doshas must then be rebalanced to assure
proper flow, energy and stability:* After the Ama is
eliminated, the blocks to maintaining proper balance
are eliminated and it becomes easy to rebalance the
Doshas.

4. *Rejuvenation — Re-enlivening the system so that it is strong
and vital:* The process of purification can take energy
and we need to replace that and strengthen the
system, so as to create more vitality, stability and flow.

The "tools" of a healing Yoga practice are actually the tools
of consciousness. We utilize consciousness or awareness to
do "the work" of purification, rather than focusing on the
digestive tract. How this happens is outlined below.

## 1. Preparation

*Softening and Loosening the Ama:* Ripening of energetic Ama occurs when we "light up" an area of the body, utilizing various Asana and Pranayama practices. By utilizing the breath and flowing that breath and our awareness to the area of the physiology requiring healing, we present the power of consciousness to energize the area holding the Ama. The key to utilizing Yoga to balance the physiology lies in its ability to re-establish the proper flow of energy and intelligence — the intelligence that organizes the balance and health of the physical body. In other words, it is the consciousness aspect of Yoga that allows us to use that method to heal. Once again let us look at a quote from the German Yoga teacher Elizabeth Haich [*Initiation*, Aurora Press, 2000]:

> Every morning at sunrise we have to assemble in the garden. We begin with physical exercises… We assume various body postures and, while doing breathing exercises, must guide our consciousness into different parts of the body. Through long and patient practice in this way we can make the entire body completely conscious, move at will, control and guide the smallest parts of the body and all internal organs. Patiently and persistently we thus develop the body into an excellent instrument.

The key to healing with Yoga is in the utilization of consciousness. The ability to guide consciousness in Yoga practices is enhanced with "breathing exercises." For this practice, various types of Pranayamas are used. One particularly useful technique is described below — "The Healing Breath." This method of breathing is key. It aids the visualizing and flowing of the breath to the area and "lights it up" in consciousness allowing the loosening process to take place.

Recall that awareness or consciousness itself is purifying. The point of Asana selection is in how that particular posture naturally pulls awareness to a particular part of the physiology. In particular, certain postures will naturally light up or enhance particular Chakras. We engage in a warm-up of the physical being, basing the Asana selection on the Chakra involved. (We determine the Chakra through the assessment methods of Ayurveda — particularly using pulse diagnosis to determine the Dosha, Subdosha and Chakra needing attention.) We then select a posture for the Chakra involved that will allow us to flow *Prana,* or subtle energy (consciousness) to the Chakra via the Healing Breath. This is done to loosen the energetic, emotional and mental Ama blocking the full functioning of that particular Chakra. Recall that the Chakras control the Subdoshas and the Doshas and have far-reaching effects on healing throughout the body, not just in the location of the Chakra.

Remember, though, that this is only the beginning. What makes Yoga effective in healing is the inner work that is done in the posture, not the posture itself. The posture is only there to turn the awareness to that Chakra or area of the body. This is why Patanjali emphasizes also that Asana be "pleasant steadiness" — **Sthira sukham asanam.** If we are to do the inner work that allows the removal of old traumas and stresses, of old emotions and cellular memories, then we must be able to stay in the posture for long periods of time. *And* the posture must be pleasant, so that it is not distracting us from going inward and exploring the energies and memories that are associated with that area of the body.

Much of this inner work is facilitated with the Healing Breath. This special Pranayama technique enhances the flow of consciousness and energy to a particular area of the body. This lights up and softens the area and greatly enhances the process.

## *The Healing Breath — Physical Mechanics*

It is well-known that increasing the pressure in the thorax creates an immediate response by the heart and the autonomic nervous system. When the blood leaves the heart as a pulse wave in the aorta, it is under high pressure, around 120mm Hg usually. When it returns to the heart it is usually around just 10mm Hg. When we increase pressure in the thorax, as when we bear down (like when having a bowel movement), this causes the return of blood to the heart to slow. When we bear down, the heart senses that it is not full and the autonomic nervous system sends out a stimulus to the parasympathetic nervous system to slow down the heart and wait a bit before the next heartbeat, so that the heart chamber can fill. Cardiologists use this "Valsalva Maneuver" to assess the heart's response and to hear more clearly the closing of the valves of the heart. They also use it sometimes to stop certain types of arrhythmias.

When we do the Healing Breath, we are stimulating the parasympathetic nervous system. This is the opposite of the sympathetic nervous system, which is responsible for the "fight or flight" response. The parasympathetic nervous system creates a relaxation response.

In addition, there is another mechanical aspect to the healing breath, important for both healing and for the development of consciousness. Normally, the pulse wave from the ejection of blood into the aorta shakes the entire body. When that wave hits the bifurcation of the aorta (where it splits into the two blood vessels that go down each leg), the pulse wave slamming against the split creates a shock wave that echoes back to the heart. Normally this shock wave is out of sync with the pulse wave coming out of the heart from the next beat. But when we slow the heart with the healing breath or during deep meditation, the slight pause for the next heartbeat allows the two waves to come into perfect sync — at 7 cycles per second. This just happens to be the frequency at which the Earth's magnetic field oscillates. In this manner, it is thought by some that we are actually able to synchronize ourselves with the Earth's magnetic vibration.

## The Healing Breath — Subtle Mechanics

In order to pull healing energy into the body from the higher energies that surround us, we must ground these energies into the physical vehicle. This is done by pulling the *Prana* (breath) down the channel of the spine known as the *Shushumna*. This happens spontaneously on the inhale of the Healing Breath. In order to ground the energy from the higher vibration into the physical we must pull it down into the first three Chakras. These are the energy centers most connected with healing the physical body.

In particular, the 1st and 2nd Chakras are important. We breathe on the exhale from the center of the 2nd Chakra with support coming from the 1st. This is important for healing because it is where our physical power resides — in our base (1st Chakra) and in our feeling sense (2nd Chakra). As many healing issues are intimately intertwined with emotional issues, the flow from the 2nd Chakra becomes even more important.

Also, it is important to note that the 2nd Chakra relates to the water element and the ability to flow emotional energy and bliss in the body. As we practice the Healing Breath, we will often notice in increase in heat in the abdomen and then an ability to direct this warmth and energy to specific areas, as we imagine the exhaled breath traveling from the abdomen to a specific part of the body (such as a painful elbow). By directing the Healing Breath from the abdomen to specific areas of the body, we bring more consciousness and awareness to that part of the body, thereby creating healing.

## The Healing Breath — The Practice

Described here are some instructions to give a more concrete idea of this type of Pranayama. It is hard to learn this properly from a book. The instructions are presented to give you the concept of how it is done, not to substitute for instruction from a teacher.

1. Put your right hand on the abdomen two finger-widths below the navel.

2. As you inhale slowly, rather than raising the chest, start with expanding the abdomen, pushing the abdomen against your hand, then filling the chest.

3. Hold the breath for a couple of seconds.

4. Exhale very slowly, with your throat almost completely closed (as if making a noise like DarthVader in movie *Star Wars*), *pushing your abdomen against your hand.* This last point is counter-intuitive as your initial tendency will be to pull the abdomen in, rather than pushing it out against your hand. You should feel a slight pressure in your abdomen and chest, as you exhale in this manner.

5. Imagine the breath flowing down to your $2^{nd}$ Chakra as you inhale and then coming from the $2^{nd}$ Chakra as you exhale.

Utilizing the Healing Breath and directing the flow to the area of the body helps to re-establish the flow and balance in that area of the body. Directing the breath to a Chakra that is out of balance also creates a profound effect both on the Chakra and on the Subdoshas and Doshas that are associated with that Chakra.

## 2. Purification

*Eliminating Ama from the system:* If we do proper preparation, the purification process happens naturally. When we are inward with our attention (facilitated by having our eyes closed), after we let the Healing Breath go, we return to our normal breathing. Putting our attention on the area in question will naturally create some purification. This can range from simply a thought to a complex dreamlike series of images or memories. At times, these can run in fast motion, if we are passive enough and allow them to come naturally, having the subtle intention to release whatever is stored in that area of the body.

We do not have to force purification. It happens naturally through the power of consciousness. Just attending to the area of the body is sufficient. We do not have to strain or stretch or force. We just have to turn our attention inward and rest it easily on the area or Chakra in question.

At times the release will come with great emotion. But most of the time, it will come with either images or thoughts. The thoughts themselves can be rather mundane. We don't really pay much attention to them, unless we can clearly distinguish an intuitive message from a mundane thought. Individuals will at times, if they are intuitive, receive additional guidance in the silence of this stage of the process. But for most, the stress that comes out is already a conglomeration of many experiences and not worth much consideration or analysis. Just like most dreams, the theme may be relevant, but most of the details are chaotic distortions.

This process takes place naturally, if we allow it. If we try to force it to happen, we can drive the Ama deeper just as when we are too aggressive and forceful with Panchakarma (physical purification techniques). This is where the process of effortless, mantra-based meditation can actually enhance the practice of Yoga. When one is used to turning inward without effort and letting go, then the purification phase is easier to do, because there is nothing *to do*, except turn our attention to the area of the body in question.

## 3. Rebalancing
*The Doshas must then be rebalanced to assure proper flow, energy and stability:* The rebalancing step involves once again lighting up the region with the breath. Until we are adept at running

subtle energy to specific areas of the body, we do this practice while visualizing the breath as an energy or light coming from the 2nd Chakra. All of the 72,000 Nadis, or subtle channels of the body, run through the 2nd Chakra, making it the major controller of energy flows in the body. The Healing Breath takes advantage of this. While not usually taught in most Yoga classes in the United States, it is known in the esoteric Yoga tradition and also in most systems of martial arts.

Once we have re-enlivened the area in question with the Healing Breath, we must then go about rebalancing this area. This requires a reorganization of the subtle energies in that region of the body. That reorganization take place through altering the qualities that are unfolding out of consciousness. Consciousness at these very subtle levels is organized via vibration or primordial sounds. Utilizing special sounds, or *mantras,* we are able to influence the way consciousness manifests into qualities that ultimately affect the human body.

For example, suppose we have an imbalance that is creating knee pain. The Ayurvedic practitioner determines from the pulse and other assessment procedures that, in this particular individual, Vata Dosha is at the root of this problem. Specifically, let's suppose that it is Apana Subdosha and the 1st Chakra that seem out of balance in the pulse. In order to correct the imbalance, the practitioner would prescribe a sound for the 1st Chakra that would also affect Apana Vata. In addition, the practitioner would look for the primary element (Mahabhuta) that is out of balance. Suppose in this case the Mahabhuta that is out of balance is air. Air has dried out the lubrication in the knee, so the joint is not protected from the impacts it sustains. In order to correct this situation, the Ayurvedic practitioner would select the sound that is associated with the Water Mahabhuta to counter the Air effect and create greater lubrication in the joint. The sound for the 1st Chakra would be combined with the sound for the Mahabhuta Water, forming a mantra of two syllables that would be used to rebalance the flow of subtle energies in the 1st Chakra and the knee.

While the mantra selection is important, the mantra is useless without the proper technique for using it. The mantra must be used to "ascend" to pure consciousness. In other words it must be used at a very subtle quiet level of the mind and carry us toward pure consciousness. It is the vehicle we use to transcend thought and enter into the silence of pure consciousness. This practice is much easier for those who have been trained in an effortless mantra-based meditation, such as Natural Meditation, Transcendental Meditation or Primordial Sound Meditation.

The best way to understand the importance of the proper use of the mantra is by analogy. Using a mantra on the gross level of the mind is like stirring the water on the surface of the ocean — it has a marginal effect. Stir the ocean floor, and it creates a tidal wave.

Each sound creates in consciousness a pattern of light as it alters the energy flow. This is actually where the design originated for the sacred alphabets, such as Sanskrit or Hebrew — they were perceived by sages invoking the sound at a subtle level of the mind. These symbols can also be used to "ascend" or "transcend" and evoke similar effects (a healing light effect). Adept Ayurvedic Yoga practitioners use both the mantra and its symbol. By energetically injecting these into the Chakra in question, a profound and dynamic effect is created. The Doshas and Subdoshas are rebalanced at their subtlest level.

The process of rebalancing involves lighting up the area with the Healing Breath, then using the appropriate mantra internally with attention to the appropriate Chakra and then transcending on the sound and light of the mantra. The rest of the rebalancing process is completed automatically by Nature itself.

## 4. Rejuvenation

*Re-enlivening the system so that it is strong and vital:* When we have been utilizing the Healing Breath, we have been running energies from the 2nd Chakra, either consciously or through visualizing this flow as light. The reason for utilizing the 2nd Chakra in this manner does not simply originate from the idea that all the Nadis flow through it. Those familiar with Patanjali will recognize that he pointed out special abilities associated with the 2nd Chakra. As MSI writes in his translation of Patanjali's Yoga Sutras [*Enlightenment*, The Ishaya Foundation Publishing Company]:

> The seven Chakras are subtle energy centers scattered along the cerebrospinal axis that control various bodily functions and are associated with certain abilities. From focusing on the navel Chakra while resonating with Ascendant [transcendental] Consciousness comes complete knowledge of the body, for all the subtle energy currents (known as Nadis) that control the physical functioning of the body pass through this Chakra. Mastery of that gives the ability to see all the internal organs and all the bodily systems; from this direct perception comes the ability to heal any area of the body that is damaged, diseased or aged.

In order to rejuvenate, we once again use the Healing Breath to flow energy from the 2nd Chakra to the area. After doing so for a few minutes, we let go of the breath and turn our awareness to the 2nd Chakra and then we let go of that. If an image of the internal aspect of the body comes, as mentioned by Patanjali, we let it come. If it doesn't, we don't force it. In either case, after we let go, we then turn our attention to the 4th Chakra and allow ourselves to feel the love and bliss that resides there. With gentle intention we send that bliss to the area of the body needing attention.

With this rejuvenation phase, we are able to complete the process that mirrors the purification process in Panchakarma. With a heart filled with gratitude and the knowledge that the healing is done, we can then move on to the process for which we have ultimately been preparing — meditation. With this process we connect much deeper in meditation and heal much faster and evolve at the fastest rate.

## THE PROCESS

It is impossible to do justice to this method and this process of maximizing the healing effects of Yoga in a book. To use this Ayurvedic Yoga obviously requires some training and re-orientation from much of what is being taught currently as Yoga. The full process actually involves more details than have been presented here, but the main concepts have been elucidated. Selection of postures for the appropriate level of student, understanding the techniques and guiding students through the process — and, most important, being able to get feedback and know how to guide the student's experience — all take some level of training. But the principles apply universally and are presented here to enhance a greater understanding of Yoga and Ayurveda. They provide a direction for practice and a knowledge of how to optimize the practice of Yoga for healing. They create the potential for maximal healing, maximal preparation for meditation, and they satisfy the sincere seeker's search for the real Yogic healing art.

# Yoga and Ayurveda

*Chapter 7*

# Health

Health is wholeness, the unity of the self with the field of consciousness. As abstract and intellectual as this understanding can be, the reality is that it affords the full development of the heart and love, and it develops the love that can heal all. Health, the real wholeness, allows for the full evolution, growth and development of the individual. This brings the full development of the heart and the bliss. Sushruta, the famous Ayurvedic surgeon who lived in approximately 220 B.C., gave this definition of health:

> He whose Doshas (physiologic functions) are in balance, whose appetite is good, whose Dhatus (tissue layers) are functioning normally, whose Malas (body wastes) are in balance, and whose body, mind and senses remain full of bliss is called a healthy person.

Notice the emphasis on bliss in his definition. When the full development occurs, the mind and senses do remain full of bliss, and in that bliss healing is automatic. Love and bliss and health all go hand in hand. It is to that wholeness that we must aspire, for the rewards are far greater than we can imagine.

**Love and Bliss**
The long-forgotten separation we have had from that wholeness makes it seem unreal. The event is so, so long ago, we have no concept, no knowledge of how being separate is an illusion. The heart knows. The heart always unites. It always yearns for unity. It seeks commonality. It seeks to find its complement and merge back into the bliss of Oneness. In the heart we know there is an escape from the torture of the mind, of the ego. In the heart we find freedom, and in love we find ourselves getting lost. So many are afraid of losing themselves in love. We don't really lose ourselves in love. We

find our real selves. So many fear they will give up what they have and what they are, so strong is the desire for love, so overwhelming the experience.

What is there to give up? What is there to be lost? Just the trail of concepts of ourselves. Just the cage of the ego... This is what is usually lost in love. But mostly we fear that we will lose control. Fear and control have no place in the temple of love. We are to know this: We each carry a divine spark and will necessarily tread our own divine path, whether it is sooner or later. And that path leads to love.

For most of us, the fear of losing ourselves in love is unfounded. It is the ego's expression of its need for control. In love, the ego is lost. In love, all sense of separateness and isolation disappears, and we rejoice in knowing that we are part of something greater, some greater whole that is so much more than the sum of its parts. It is a hint of the higher consciousness and higher development to come.

Even the energy flows in the body are affected, in that they are merged. From the physical, to the energetic, to the emotional, to the spiritual — love creates a ground-shaking transformation of the self into a greater Self. For most people, this transcendental experience is their *only* escape from the confines of the ego, of the limited sense of isolated self. They have no experience of the power of meditation and Yogic healing. No wonder the physical act of love has such a draw and fascination for the human being. It is not a matter of procreation, as it is for the animals. It is a beautiful release from the prison of the ego.

When the beautiful unity of love becomes confused with sacrifice, then trouble begins. Sacrifice has come to mean a loss, a giving up of something for someone else. Here the ego feels a pain at having to give up something, while at the same time it congratulates itself on being "good" and doing the "loving" thing. The ego pushes on and attempts to give that which it does not have, in order to feel good about itself.

Sacrifice means to make sacred. You make something sacred by infusing Divinity into it. Then it is Divine, and it is sacred. You can only give that which you have. And you can only make something sacred when you have the fullness of the Divinity, the bliss of Being within you. There is no loss in real sacrifice because real love flows effortlessly and only increases in bliss as it expands and flows out to others. It is in fullness that we truly have something to give. When we strain to give, the stress of the strain taints the gift. When we have captured bliss in our awareness, then we have ability to allow love to flow out without loss, creating more and more joy — more and more bliss.

Contact with the field of bliss, the field of pure consciousness (the field of pure love) is the most important way to develop the capacity for true sacrifice. In that experience we infuse the mind with Being. Then we have the full capability to make anything sacred. Then we can "sacrifice" without loss. In doing for someone else, we know we are doing it for ourselves. For in the experience of the field of pure consciousness, we come to know that we are not our isolated concept of ourselves. We have as much joy in giving to others as we have in giving to ourselves — even more, perhaps — because the joy we experience in the delight of the other is so much more interesting than our own.

In real love, nothing is lost. Only the ego is left behind. That incredible rush — that bliss that we experience when falling in love, when being in the arms of another, when finding the rapture of being cherished and desired by another — that is an experience that can rip us away from the mind's old patterns and plunge us deep into the bliss that resides in the center of our being. And that bliss can heal the worst of wounds and the deadliest of diseases.

Capturing the bliss and living a life of love and health is not reserved for the experience of falling in love. It is available to anyone at anytime. It does not depend on finding "the right person." It does not depend on being with someone else. It only requires a way to go deep within, past the mental chatter, past the subconscious mind, past the waves of feelings into the depths of the ocean of pure awareness, pure consciousness, pure bliss.

That is our nature. That is our inheritance. That is where our health resides. That is what we must connect with in order to have perfect health. And that is what Yoga and Ayurveda are all about.

# Yoga and Ayurveda

*Appendix*

RESOURCES

# Resources

TRAINING IN AYURVEDIC YOGA / NATURAL MEDITATION / THE HEALING BREATH

New World Ayurveda
1522 State Street
Santa Barbara, CA 93101
888-833-2108
www.newworldayurveda.com

AYURVEDIC HEALTH PRACTITIONER'S TRAINING

New World Ayurveda
1522 State Street
Santa Barbara, CA 93101
888-833-2108
www.newworldayurveda.com

AYURVEDIC CONSULTATIONS

Paul Dugliss, M.D.
1522 State Street
Santa Barbara, CA 93101
805-248-7088
www.drdugliss.com

# About the Author

**Paul Dugliss, M.D.** practices Ayurvedic Medicine and Internal Medicine in Santa Barbara, California. He is the former director of the Oakwood Healthcare System's Complementary & Alternative Medicine Center in Westland, Michigan. A student of Ayurvedic Medicine since the 1980s, he trained both in this country and abroad. Dr. Dugliss also has training in acupuncture and Traditional Chinese Medicine, as well as a masters degree in Clinical and Counseling Psychology. He is the author of several books including *Ayurveda – The Power to Heal, Enlightened Nutrition, Capturing the Bliss – Ayurveda and the Yoga of Emotions,* and *The Myth of Cholesterol.*

CPSIA information can be obtained at www.ICGtesting.com
Printed in the USA
BVOW10s0647121115

426741BV00009BA/38/P

9 780972 123327